Glaucoma Identification
and Co-management

ET

Commissioning Editor: Robert Edwards
Development Editor: Kim Benson
Production Manager: Caroline Horton/Frances Affleck
Design: Stewart Larking

Glaucoma
Identification and
Co-management

Edited by

David F Edgar BSc, MCOptom

Professor of Clinical Optometry, Department of Optometry and Visual Science, City University, London, UK

Alicja R Rudnicka MSc, PhD, MCOptom

Senior Research Fellow in Epidemiology and Medical Statistics, Division of Community Health Sciences, St George's, University of London, London, UK

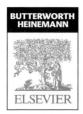

EDINBURGH LONDON NEW YORK OXFORD PHILADELPHIA ST LOUIS SYDNEY TORONTO 2007

BUTTERWORTH
HEINEMANN
ELSEVIER

First published 2007

The rights of David F Edgar and Alicja R Rudnicka to be identified as authors of
this work have been asserted by them in accordance with the Copyright, Designs
and Patents Act 1988.

ISBN-13: 9780750637824
ISBN-10: 0-7506-3782-X

British Library Cataloguing in Publication Data
A catalogue record for this book is available from the British Library.

Library of Congress Cataloging in Publication Data
A catalog record for this book is available from the Library of Congress.

Note
Knowledge and best practice in this field are constantly changing. As new
research and experience broaden our knowledge, changes in practice, treatment
and drug therapy may become necessary or appropriate. Readers are advised to
check the most current information provided (i) on procedures featured or (ii)
by the manufacturer of each product to be administered, to verify the
recommended dose or formula, the method and duration of administration, and
contraindications. It is the responsibility of the practitioner, relying on their own
experience and knowledge of the patient, to make diagnoses, to determine
dosages and the best treatment for each individual patient, and to take all
appropriate safety precautions. To the fullest extent of the law, neither the
Publisher nor the Editors assume any liability for any injury and/or damage to
persons or property arising out of or related to any use of the material contained
in this book.
The Publisher

ELSEVIER your source for books,
journals and multimedia
in the health sciences
www.elsevierhealth.com

Working together to grow
libraries in developing countries

www.elsevier.com | www.bookaid.org | www.sabre.org

ELSEVIER   BOOK AID International   Sabre Foundation

The
publisher's
policy is to use
paper manufactured
from sustainable forests

Printed in China

Contents

Preface

The origins of *Glaucoma Identification and Co-management* can be traced back to the introduction in 1996 of the first two Certificate courses for registered Optometrists run jointly by City University and Moorfields Eye Hospital: Diabetic Shared Care and Glaucoma Shared Care. In 1999 *Diabetic Eye Disease Identification and Co-management* was published with chapters written by contributors to the Diabetic Shared Care course, and it is with great pleasure that we introduce the sister book written by contributors to the Glaucoma course. This course is now run annually by City University.

There are approximately 250,000 sufferers from Primary Open Angle Glaucoma (POAG) in the UK, with possibly a similar number remaining undiagnosed in the community. POAG patients now represent 25–30% of the outpatient load of ophthalmology departments in the UK, and this outpatient burden will increase as life expectancy increases and as our methods of detection of glaucoma become more sensitive.

A general finding from population based surveys is that approximately 50% of people found to have glaucoma were previously undiagnosed, hence the role of general practitioners, optometrists and technicians as primary screeners has been investigated. Consensus is yet to be reached on the most effective way to screen for glaucoma, and at present there is no satisfactory test that would be suitable for mass screening for glaucoma. Evidence on the efficacy of treatments to prevent further deterioration of visual function in glaucoma is only just emerging in the literature. For these reasons population screening for POAG is probably unjustified in Westernised populations.

Glaucoma will place demands on the NHS that will require innovative approaches to patient management, including the development and refinement of co-management/shared-care schemes. *Glaucoma Identification and Co-management* aims to provide the background knowledge needed by optometrists embarking on co-management/shared-care of POAG and to reinforce the knowledge of those already involved in co-management/shared-care practice. While the majority of readers will be registered optometrists, the book will also serve as a valuable reference work for students of optometry. The book provides detailed methods of clinical examination techniques and their interpretation together with a detailed description of the histopathology, physiology and visual functional changes in glaucoma. Therefore, it may be of use to general practitioners and medical students with an interest in glaucoma, as well as other healthcare professionals with an interest in the identification and co-management of glaucoma.

Co-management/shared-care schemes require a combination of skills from several disciplines – notably ophthalmology and optometry – and these professions are well represented among our authors. We also have a contribution from a pharmacist as pharmacy is another profession with a key role to play in the management of patients suffering from glaucoma. We are most grateful to all our authors, who have worked together so diligently to produce this book.

David F Edgar   Alicja R Rudnicka

Contributor List

Christopher Bentley
Visiting Professor of Ophthalmology, Middlesex University; Honorary Senior Lecturer, Imperial College, London; Consultant Ophthalmic Surgeon, Central Middlesex Hospital, London, UK

Jill Bloom
Medicines Information Pharmacist, Department of Pharmacology, Moorfields Eye Hospital, London, UK

Philip Bloom
Visiting Professor of Ophthalmology, Middlesex University; Honorary Senior Lecturer, Imperial College, London; Consultant Ophthalmic Surgeon, Western Eye Hospital and Hillingdon Hospital, London, UK

Yvonne Delaney
Ophthalmologist, Eye Department, Mater Misericordiae Hospital, Dublin, Ireland

David F Edgar
Professor of Clinical Optometry, Department of Optometry and Visual Science, City University, London, UK

John G Flanagan
Professor, School of Optometry, University of Waterloo; Professor, Department of Ophthalmology and Vision Sciences, University of Toronto; Senior Scientist, Toronto Western Research Institute, University Health Network, Ontario, Canada

Robert Harper
Consultant Optometrist, Manchester Royal Eye Hospital; Honorary Senior Lecturer, University of Manchester, Manchester, UK

David B Henson
Professor of Ophthalmology and Vision Sciences, University of Manchester, Manchester, UK

Peng T Khaw
Professor of Glaucoma and Ocular Healing, Paediatric Glaucoma Unit, Moorfields Eye Hospital and Wound Healing Research Unit, Institute of Ophthalmology, London, UK

John G Lawrenson
Professor of Clinical Visual Science, Department of Optometry and Visual Science, City University, London, UK

Colm O'Brien
Professor of Ophthalmology, University College Dublin, Mater Hospital, Dublin, Ireland

Christopher G Owen
Senior Lecturer in Epidemiology, Division of Community Health Sciences, St. George's, University of London, London, UK

C Lisa Prokopich
Lecturer, School of Optometry, University of Waterloo; Head, Ocular Health Clinic, School of Optometry, University of Waterloo; Head, Freeport Hospital Vision Centre, Kitchener, Ontario, Canada

Simon J A Rankin
Consultant Ophthalmic Surgeon, Ophthalmology Department, Royal Hospitals, Belfast, Northern Ireland, UK

Alicja Rudnicka
*Senior Research Fellow in Epidemiology and
Medical Statistics, Division of Community Health
Sciences, St George's, University of London, London,
UK*

Peter Shah
*Consultant Ophthalmologist, Birmingham and
Midland Eye Centre, Birmingham, UK*

Paul G D Spry
*Head Optometrist, Departments of Shared Care
and Visual Electrophysiology, Bristol Eye Hospital,
Bristol, UK*

David Thomson
*Professor of Optometry and Visual Science,
Department of Optometry and Visual Science,
City University, London, UK*

Mark R Wilkins
*Consultant Ophthalmologist, Moorfields Eye
Hospital, London, UK*

Sarah J Wilson
*Glaucoma Fellow, Eye and Ear Clinic, Royal
Victoria Hospital, Belfast, Northern Ireland, UK*

Chapter 1

Epidemiology of primary open angle glaucoma

Alicja R Rudnicka and Christopher G Owen

GENERAL EPIDEMIOLOGICAL PRINCIPLES

Epidemiology is the study of the incidence, distribution and determinants of disease in human populations with a view to identifying their causes and bringing about their prevention.

A cause of a disease is a factor that is associated with the disease so that if the intensity or prevalence of the factor in a population is changed, the incidence of the disease also changes.

Wald (2004)[1]

Epidemiology is concerned with examining groups of individuals with the intention of identifying risk factors that are present *before* the disease is clinically manifest and thereby identify a cause (or causes) for the disease. Once a cause is identified it may then be possible to bring about prevention of disease by removal or modification of the causal factor. An example of a study to investigate the epidemiology of a disease would involve examining a population sample of people who do not yet have the disease of interest and measuring various risk factors over time (such as age, social class, smoking status, alcohol consumption, blood pressure) and then waiting to see who develops the disease in later life.

The method of analysis is concerned with examining differences in the pattern of the risk factors in those who develop and those who do not develop the disease of interest. This study design is called a cohort study, from which we can also quantify the burden (e.g. prevalence and incidence—see below) of the disease. A simpler form of population study is a cross-sectional study (i.e. a survey or prevalence study), which involves measuring risk factors and disease outcomes at the same point in time; there is no long-term follow-up of the sample. However, unlike a cohort design, disease incidence cannot be ascertained, and one cannot be certain whether a risk factor associated with a disease caused the disease or occurred as a consequence of the disease. Another type of epidemiological study identifies people who already have the disease (i.e. cases) and a suitable control group (i.e. people who do not have the disease but are representative of the population from which cases of the disease have arisen) and involves comparing risk factors of interest between both groups. This is called a case–control study, and although this design does not give a measure of disease burden, and cannot always distinguish whether a risk factor(s) was present before the disease developed, case–control studies are useful in the study of rare diseases, such as glaucoma. These different epidemiological study designs have advantages and disadvantages that are not within the scope of this chapter. However, the reason for describing these study designs is to highlight some of the different types of epidemiological study used in this chapter to assimilate the evidence concerning the burden of glaucoma and potential risk factors for glaucoma.

Prevalence (also referred to as point prevalence) is the proportion of people in a defined population who have the disease of interest in a defined time period. It is simply a proportion or a percentage, e.g. disease A has a prevalence of 1% in persons aged 45–55 years of age, and an alternative way to express this is 10 per 1000 population aged 45–55 years of age.

Incidence is the number of *new* cases of a disease occurring in a defined population over a specified period of time. Incidence rate is the rate of disease, e.g. disease A has an incidence of 1 per 10000 per year in persons over 40 years of age.

Risk factor is any factor measured either in an individual or in a group of individuals that is associated with the risk of a disease.

1.1 GENERAL DEFINITIONS OF THE GLAUCOMAS

The glaucomas are a group of ocular diseases that may cause characteristic progressive changes in the optic nerve head, visual field loss, or both.[2] Glaucomas can be subdivided into primary conditions in which the mechanism for the disease is unknown, and secondary conditions where the glaucoma is secondary to another ocular or systemic disease. Secondary glaucoma typically results in raised intraocular pressure (IOP) secondary to, for example, cataract, trauma, uveitis and disorders affecting the drainage and structure of the anterior chamber angle.

Primary and secondary glaucomas can be further subdivided into open angle and angle closure (also called closed or narrow angle glaucoma), which directly relates to whether the anterior chamber angle and the region for aqueous drainage is open or narrowed. Chapter 2 describes in detail aqueous production and drainage and Chapter 4 describes the clinical examination of the anterior chamber angle and quantification of its structure.

Primary open angle glaucoma (POAG) has an adult onset, is usually bilateral and produces characteristic changes in the optic nerve head or visual field (see Chapters 3, 5, 7 and 9) and these changes may be in the presence or absence of elevated IOP. In more advanced stages of POAG, patients become aware of the visual deficits. Although IOP can be raised in POAG it is not a prerequisite of POAG. Historically there was a great deal of emphasis on IOP in the glaucoma literature and this led to a misunderstanding that heightened IOP was synonymous with POAG. There is considerable overlap in the levels of IOP in people with and without glaucomatous optic neuropathy. The clinical definition of POAG does not depend on the eye having an eye pressure above a given IOP, for example, 21 mmHg, but treatment of POAG is primarily concerned with reducing IOP (see

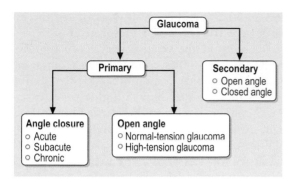

Fig. 1.1 Classification of the glaucomas.

Chapters 10–12). Chapter 8 provides more detailed information on the measurement of and factors that influence the variability of IOP in normal and glaucomatous populations and gives guidelines for referral of patients.

A large proportion of the glaucoma literature is focused on IOP and this has led to further subgroups, defined on the basis of IOP (see Fig 1.1).

- POAG, which is subdivided into:
  - normal-tension glaucoma (formerly called low tension glaucoma), which includes those with glaucomatous optic neuropathy but with IOP within the 'normal range'
  - 'high-tension' or 'classical' glaucoma, being POAG with raised IOP.
- Ocular hypertension; those with raised IOP (usually IOP above 21 mmHg) but no optic nerve damage or visual field loss.

In American and European populations between 2% and 10% of people will have IOP above 21 mmHg, and prospective studies suggest that of these only 1–3% per year develop glaucoma.[3–7] Therefore most patients with ocular hypertension do not go on to develop glaucoma. However, very high IOPs require treatment because of the risk of central retinal vein occlusion.

These subgroups of POAG are attempts to split the population into specific groups when in reality there is a continuous spectrum of risk factors in people. The correlation between IOP and POAG is analogous to the relationship between blood pressure and cardiovascular disease; there is a great deal of overlap in the distribution of blood pressure values of people who have cardiovascular disease and those who do not. There is no real lower safe limit below which cardiovascular disease never occurs. The overlap in blood pressure levels between affected and unaffected individuals is one of the main reasons why screening for cardiovascular disease by measuring blood pressure is not an effective screening test. The same problem arises in screening the population for glaucoma by the measurement of IOP alone.

This chapter focuses on the epidemiology of POAG, since in the UK and other European populations it accounts for the vast majority of the glaucomas.

1.2 PREVALENCE OF PRIMARY OPEN ANGLE GLAUCOMA

There are many population-based surveys on the prevalence of glaucoma. Unfortunately many of the older publications did not differentiate between POAG and primary angle closure glaucoma (PACG). However, the latter is far less common than POAG in white populations and those of European descent[8–13] and therefore the estimates are likely to reflect mainly cases of POAG. In white people 75–95% of primary glaucoma is open angle whereas in Asians the findings are more variable with 30–90% of primary glaucoma being angle closure. The population sampling procedures in the prevalence studies were of reasonable quality but few studies conducted visual field examination on all subjects. Visual field testing was typically performed on 'high-risk' individuals such as those with suspicious optic discs or raised IOP. Unfortunately this leads to biased estimates of the numbers of subjects with glaucoma because it is now generally accepted that approximately half of patients with clinically defined glaucoma have IOP in the 'normal' range and, in addition, the IOP can vary considerably within an individual. Hence such study designs were likely to have missed cases of glaucoma that had IOPs within what would have arbitrarily been defined as the 'normal range' and so underestimated the number with glaucoma. An interesting observation in nearly all the population surveys is that about half of the cases of POAG detected at the time of survey were previously undiagnosed.

1.2.1 GEOGRAPHICAL AND ETHNIC DISTRIBUTION OF PRIMARY GLAUCOMA

Table 1.1 summarises the prevalence of POAG and PACG from some of the larger population-based studies[9,10,12,14–42]. Although the methods of testing and sampling vary from one study to another they give an idea of the relative prevalence in different populations. The prevalence for POAG ranges from 0.03% in China to 8.76% in St Lucia; most of the studies in Table 1.1 are in people aged 30 years or more. The relative prevalence of PACG and POAG differs dramatically according to race and age. In Europeans, Africans and North Americans POAG is the most predominant form of glaucoma.

The prevalence of POAG in those aged over 40 years in white people from Europe, America and Australia of comparable age groups is of the same order (approximately 1–3%), whereas black populations in the Caribbean and the USA have higher prevalence in similar age groups. Currently the highest prevalence of POAG is reported in black populations of the Caribbean, particularly St Lucia and Barbados, (~7–9%), with slightly lower prevalence (3–4%) in black Africans from Baltimore, London and other parts of Africa.[12,14–18] The Baltimore Eye Study directly compared the prevalence in white and black people from the same geographical location, and the age-adjusted rates were 4.3 times higher in Black Americans compared with White Americans.[12] The age of onset of POAG appears to be earlier in Africans than in white Europeans and seems to progress more rapidly and may be more resistant to IOP reduction therapy. Interestingly, primary glaucoma was not found in pure-blooded New Zealand Maoris and was uncommon in Australians of aboriginal origin;[43,44] an explanation for these findings remains unclear. A recent systematic review and meta-analysis of 46 cross-sectional studies, that included 2509 cases of POAG, found that Blacks had the highest prevalence of POAG at all ages compared to Whites and Asians.[45] The prevalence of POAG in those aged 50–59 years was estimated to be 4.6% in Blacks, 0.8% in Whites and 1% in Asians; in those aged 60–69 years the estimates were respectively 7.2%, 1.6% and 1.6%; and over 70 years of age the estimates were 16%, 6% and 3% respectively.

Variability in the relative prevalence of PACG and POAG in studies conducted in Chinese and Asian (Mongoloid) communities exists, although most of these studies show a higher prevalence of PACG compared with studies carried out in European, American and African populations (Table 1.1). Japan appears to be the exception, where the prevalence of PACG is extremely low (0.08%), and much lower than the prevalence of POAG (2.53%).[21] Japan is also unusual because the majority of the POAG cases have IOPs within the 'normal' range (2% with 'normal' IOP and 0.53% with raised IOP).[21] A recent survey in Japan found 92% of patients with POAG had IOP below 21 mmHg.[27] Also, mean levels of IOP in Japan have been shown to be lower than in European populations.[21] Conversely, in India the prevalence of PACG has been shown to be far greater than the prevalence of POAG (4.3% versus 0.4%, respectively).[23] The Mamre in South Africa are a mixed racial group with ancestors from south-east Asia and later migrants who came from east Africa and western Europe, and the prevalences of POAG and PACG are similar in the Mamre population.[33]

Across different ethnic groups there are marked variations in glaucoma prevalence. This may partly be explained by differences in survey methodology, but may also allude to different mechanisms for glaucoma or genetic susceptibility.

1.3 INCIDENCE OF PRIMARY OPEN ANGLE GLAUCOMA

There are fewer studies of glaucoma incidence. Extrapolations from the Framingham and Ferndale prevalence studies gave a 5-year incidence of 0.2% at age 55 years, increasing to 1% at 75 years (equivalent to 4 per 10 000 per year and 20 per 10 000 per year respectively).[13,30] Bengtsson[46] reported 24 per 10 000 per year in Sweden in those over 55 years of age. In the Melbourne Visual Impairment study the incidence was reported as 12 per 10 000 per year in those aged 60–69, 28 per 10 000 per year in the 70–79 age group and 82 per 10 000 per year in those aged over 80 years.[7] Longitudinal follow-up of the Barbados Eye Study[6] showed a

Table 1.1 **Population-based prevalence surveys of glaucoma by ethnic group***

Ethnic origin	Author(s)	Year	Name/location	Age group	Sample size	POAG (%)	PACG (%)	OHT (%)
Black	Mason et al[14]	1989	St Lucia, West Indies	30–70+	1679	8.76	—	—
	Tielsch et al[12]	1991	Baltimore, USA	40–80+	2395	4.18	—	—
	Leske et al[15]	1994	Barbados, West Indies	40–86	4498	6.8	—	—
	Wormald et al[16]	1994	London, UK	35–60+	873	3.67	—	2.18
	Buhrmann et al[17]	2000	Kongwa, East Africa	40–80+	3247	3.08	0.59	
	Rotchford et al[18]	2003	Temba, South Africa	40–97	839	3.69	0.6	
Asian	Awasthi et al[19]	1975	Agra, India	30–70+	3603	1.33	—	—
	Hu[20]	1989	Shunyi, Beijing	40+	3000	0.03	1.4	—
	Shiose et al[21]	1991	Japan	30–70+	8924	2.53	0.08	1.52
	Foster et al[22]	1996	Hovsgol, Mongolia	40–89	942	0.53	1.49	—
	Jacob et al[23]	1998	Vellore, India	30–60	972	0.41	4.32	3.09
	Foster et al[24]	2000	Singapore	40–81	1232	1.79	1.14	—
	Metheetrairut et al[25]	2002	Bangkok, Thailand	60–104	2092	2.92	2.53	—
	Ramakrishnan et al[26]	2003	Aravind, South India	40–90	5150	1.24	0.5	1.11
	Iwase et al[27]	2004	Tajimi, Japan	40–80+	3021	3.94	—	0.8
Eskimo	Arkell et al[28]	1987	Kotzebue, Alaska	15–70+	1686	0.06	0.59	—
White	Hollows et al[13]	1966	Ferndale, Wales	40–74	4231	0.47	0.09	9.38
	Bankes et al[29]	1968	Bedford, UK	20–80+	5941	0.76	0.17	3.03
	Leibowitz et al[30]	1980	Framingham, USA	<65–75+	2631	1.9	—	—
	Bengtsson[9]	1981	Dalby, Sweden	58.5–68.5	1511	0.86	0.13	0.79
	Ringvold et al[31]	1991	Norway	65–89+	1871	3.37	—	1.34
	Tielsch et al[12]	1991	Baltimore, USA	40–80+	2913	1.1	—	—
	Klein et al[32]	1992	Beaver Dam, USA	43–75+	4926	2.11	—	—
	Coffey et al[10]	1993	Roscommon, Ireland	50–80+	2186	1.88	0.09	2.97
	Salmon et al[33]	1993	Mamre, South Africa	40–70+	987	1.52	2.33	
	Dielemans et al[34]	1994	Rotterdam, Netherlands	55–75+	3062	1.11	—	—
	Leske et al[15]	1994	Barbados, West Indies	40–86	133	0.75	—	—
	Giuffre et al[35]	1995	Casteldaccia, Sicily	40–99	1062	1.22	—	2.73
	Hirvela et al[36]	1994	Oulu, Finland	70–95	500	10.4	—	—
	Mitchell et al[37]	1996	Blue Mountains, Australia	49–80+	3654	2.38	—	3.69
	Cedrone et al[38]	1997	Ponza, Italy	40–80+	1034	2.51	0.97	6
	Wensor et al[39]	1998	Melbourne, Australia	40–90+	3265	1.72	0.06	0.49
	Bonomi et al[40]	1998	Egna-Neumarkt, Italy	40–80+	4297	1.4	0.61	2.07
	Reidy et al[41]	1998	North London, UK	65–100	1547	3.04	—	—
	Quigley et al[42]	2001	Proyecto, USA	41–90+	4774	1.97	0.1	—

* In the prevalence estimates POAG includes where possible those that were classified as 'normal' tension glaucoma.
OHT, ocular hypertension; POAG, primary open angle glaucoma; PACG, primary angle closure glaucoma.

Table 1.2 Prevalence estimates of POAG according to intraocular pressure (IOP)

Baltimore Eye Study[48]		Blue Mountains Eye Study[37]	
IOP (mmHg)	Prevalence of POAG (%)	IOP (mmHg)	Prevalence of POAG (%)
16–21	1.5	12–13	0.9
22–29	8.3	22–23	5.7
≥30	25	>28	39

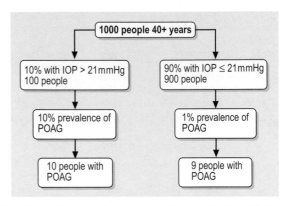

Fig. 1.2 Hypothetical example illustrating how it is possible in patients with primary open angle glaucoma (POAG) to have roughly half with raised intraocular pressure (IOP) and half with 'normal' IOP, assuming a prevalence of 10% of POAG in those with IOP above 21 mmHg and 1% in those with IOP ≤ 21 mmHg.

higher incidence in Black Caribbeans. The 4-year risk of open angle glaucoma in black participants was 2.2%, which is equivalent to 55 per 10 000 people per year. The rates were 1.2% per 4 years (30 per 10 000 per year) in those aged 40–49 years rising to 4.2% (105 per 10 000 per year) at ages 70 years or more. In the Barbados and Melbourne studies, subjects with higher IOPs at baseline were more likely to develop POAG at follow-up.[6,7]

1.4 RISK FACTORS FOR PRIMARY OPEN ANGLE GLAUCOMA

Currently several risk factors have been identified for primary open angle glaucoma but as yet the underlying cause is not known. It has been suggested that a combination of risk factors such as decreased blood flow to the optic nerve head and IOP levels that are too high in an individual may contribute to ganglion cell death. Autoimmune reactions such as increased levels of glutamate and nitric oxide have been implicated with ganglion cell death[47] but these factors have not been demonstrated to be associated with POAG in prospective epidemiological studies and so it cannot be ruled out that these factors are a consequence of rather than a cause of the disease.

1.4.1 OCULAR RISK FACTORS

Intraocular pressure

Epidemiological studies have shown that as IOP increases there is a corresponding increase in the prevalence of glaucomatous optic nerve atrophy and visual field loss.[12,48] Apart from the mechanical effect of raised IOP on the retinal nerve fibre layer and optic nerve head, other contributing factors including perfusion to the optic nerve and structural support within the lamina cribrosa have been implicated in the pathogenesis of POAG. Table 1.2 gives the prevalence estimates from two large studies according to level of IOP.

Comparing the lowest and middle IOP groups the increase in POAG prevalence with increasing IOP is approximately six-fold, and is about 16–40-fold comparing the lowest and highest IOP groups. Among patients with asymmetrical IOP, usually the eye with the higher pressure has the greater degree of cupping or visual field loss. Glaucoma is rare in eyes with IOP less than 10 mmHg. The arbitrary cut-off at 21 mmHg to define elevated IOP is a statistical concept based on the mean value (16 mmHg) plus 2 standard deviations (2×2.5 mmHg), and if the distribution of IOP followed a Gaussian distribution we would expect 2.5% of the population to have IOPs above 21 mmHg. However, the distribution of IOP is not Gaussian but positively skewed, meaning that there is a higher proportion of high IOPs than expected for a Gaussian distribution; indeed, up to approximately 10% of people have IOPs above 21 mmHg. In population-based surveys it has been found that between one-third and two-thirds of those with POAG have IOPs below 21 mmHg at screening and 20–30% of POAG patients have IOP consistently less than or equal to 21 mmHg.[10,13,30,34,35,37,48–50] Figure 1.2 is a hypo-

Fig. 1.3 Age-specific prevalence estimates from some of the larger population-based studies. BMES, Blue Mountains Eye Study[37]; Barb ES, Barbados Eye Study[15]; BES, Baltimore Eye Study (in white and black people)[12]; BDES, Beaver Dam Eye Study[32]; MSA, Mamre, South Africa[33]; RI, Roscommon, Ireland.[10]

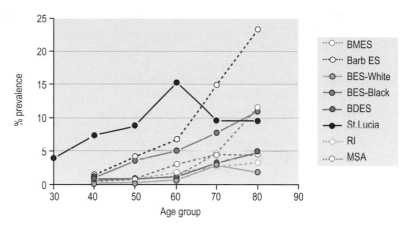

thetical example showing that if the proportion of people with IOPs above 21 mmHg is 10% and the prevalence of POAG in this group is also 10%, and the prevalence of POAG in the remaining 90% of people is 1%, then roughly half of the cases of POAG have 'normal' IOP and the other half raised IOP.

There is a continuous relationship between the level of IOP and risk of glaucoma. There is some evidence that IOP increases with age in Europeans and decreases with age in Japanese. IOP is a risk factor (not a defining causative factor) for glaucoma and lowering IOP has been shown to reduce the rate of visual field loss in some patients (see Chapters 10 and 11).

Myopia

When the association between POAG and myopia was first shown in case–control studies it was thought to be due to selection bias and not a real association. The bias was thought to arise because myopic people are more likely to attend for routine eye examinations and therefore are more likely to be screened for glaucoma compared to people without refractive errors. The consequence is that myopic people could be over-represented in glaucoma cases that are referred to clinics. For some time this association was thought to be due to this type of bias and therefore not a true association. However, recent population-based surveys have reaffirmed this association. Mitchell et al[51] found that low myopia (−1 D to less than −3 D) was associated with a doubling of the risk of glaucoma (at any age) and a three-fold increase with moderate myopia (−3 D or more myopic) compared to those

with emmetropia. This is in agreement with other studies.[52–54] The association with myopia is believed to be independent of IOP.

1.4.2 DEMOGRAPHIC AND GENETIC RISK FACTORS

Age

As shown in Table 1.1 the prevalence of POAG in those aged 40 years or more varies considerably across populations. Such differences may be due to genuine differences in prevalence, sampling errors in the estimates or differences in the methodology and definitions used to diagnose cases of POAG. Despite this variability, numerous population-based studies have found that the prevalence and incidence of POAG increases with age.[37,55–57] On average, individuals aged 70 years or older have three to four times the risk of POAG compared with 40–50-year-olds. Figure 1.3 shows the heterogeneity in prevalence estimates between some of the larger population-based studies. However, the prevalence of POAG clearly increases with age. Figure 1.3 also shows the higher prevalence among subjects of African-Caribbean origin (the St Lucia and Barbados studies) compared with other studies carried out in predominantly white populations. A meta-analysis of published surveys of POAG found an exponential increase in POAG prevalence with age that varied by racial group. In Whites the prevalence of POAG approximately doubled per decade, whereas in Blacks and Asians the prevalence of POAG increased by 60% per decade.[45]

Gender

Whether there is a gender difference in the prevalence of POAG was controversial, and studies that report gender differences may have been confounded by age. Numerous studies have found the prevalence to be higher in men,[15,30,34,41] conversely some have reported a higher prevalence in women,[9,14] whereas other studies report no gender difference in prevalence.[5,10,12,13,21,32,37,39] A meta-analysis of gender differences in POAG prevalence in Whites found that men were 1.23 times more likely than women to have POAG.[45] A similar effect was observed in Blacks and Asians. This agrees well with gender differences in the prevalence of treatment for glaucoma and ocular hypertension in the UK, reporting that males were 1.24 times more likely to receive treatment than females.[58] Despite this similarity it is still unclear whether this latter gender difference represents inequality in treatment or true differences in prevalence of disease.

Socioeconomic status, alcohol drinking and smoking

Eye problems are more prevalent in people living in relatively underprivileged areas.[41] In addition, uptake of eye examinations is low amongst unskilled socioeconomic groups.[59] Hence, those who have the least material and psychosocial resources to cope with blindness may be at substantially higher risk of glaucoma and glaucomatous visual loss.[60,61] Whether this reflects social class variations in the prevalence or incidence of POAG,[41,62] or that those from less privileged circumstances present with different stages of glaucomatous disease remains unclear;[60] further population-based studies are needed to establish the influence of socioeconomic status on POAG. Epidemiological observations are yet to show whether alcohol consumption and/or cigarette consumption, which are known to be associated with socioeconomic factors, have any discernible effect on the prevalence of POAG.[42,63] A recent systematic review and meta-analysis of four case–control studies and three cross-sectional studies found that current smokers were 1.37 times more likely to have POAG than non-smokers.[64] However, this finding was of borderline statistical

significance. More data from epidemiological studies is needed and the analysis should take into account other risk factors that are related to both the risk of POAG and smoking (e.g. age, ethnicity, socioeconomic status).[64] Past smokers had a similar risk of POAG to non-smokers.[64]

Family history

The hereditability of POAG has been calculated from twin studies to be as high as 70–80% and 98% has been reported in monozygotic twins.[65] POAG cases identified by cross-sectional survey (i.e. prevalent cases) are two to three times more likely to report a family history of glaucoma compared with controls[66–69] and four times more likely to report sibling history of glaucoma.[68] In the Rotterdam study[70] the lifetime risk of glaucoma was nine times higher in siblings and offspring of glaucoma patients than in siblings and offspring of controls (controls are individuals without glaucoma). The incidence of POAG was found to be double in those with a positive family history of POAG compared with those without a family history.[7] In summary the risk of glaucoma is stronger with sibling family history than with parental or offspring family history.

Genetics

Although a family history of glaucoma may predispose an individual to POAG, glaucoma appears to be a polygenetic disorder with no clear mendelian mode of inheritance.[71] This may well reflect the diversity of glaucomatous disease. Recently, a number of gene loci and two genes have been reported to be associated with POAG (Table 1.3).[72] The *MYOC* and *OPTN* genes are responsible for encoding the proteins myocillin and optineurin, respectively. It has been proposed that these proteins may impair or alter aqueous outflow leading to glaucomatous disease. However, the function of these proteins remains unclear. It has been estimated from studies involving ethnically diverse groups that genetic encoding mutations for myocillin production may account for 2–4% of POAG cases, and for optineurin even fewer.[73] Hence, genes identified so far are only associated with a small proportion of POAG cases. Future

Table 1.3	Genes and loci associated with POAG[72]			
Gene	Locus	Chromosome	Phenotype	Inheritance
MYOC	GLC1A	1q23-24	POAG, JOAG	AD
	GLC1B	2cen-q13	POAG	AD
	GLC1C	3q21-24	POAG	AD
	GLC1D	8p23	POAG	AD
OPTN	GLC1E	10p14-15	OAG	AD
	GLC1F	7q35-36	POAG	AD

MYOC, encodes for myocillin; OPTN, encodes for optineurin; POAG, primary open angle glaucoma; JOAG, juvenile open angle glaucoma; OAG, open angle glaucoma; AD, autosomal dominant.

work in this area may unearth more sensitive markers for POAG, but for now genetic testing for glaucoma remains a distant reality.[74] Details of genes and gene loci associated with other less common types of glaucoma, e.g. juvenile open angle glaucoma (JOAG) and congenital glaucomas are summarised elsewhere.[72–74]

1.4.3 SYSTEMIC DISEASE RISK FACTORS IN GLAUCOMA

Hypertension and diabetes

Systemic blood pressure has been related to glaucoma risk in several studies;[75–77] this may emanate from the small positive association between systolic blood pressure and IOP.[50,78] Effects on ocular perfusion pressure mean that both systemic hypertension and hypotension have been implicated as risk factors for glaucoma. This relation may alter with age,[79] perhaps resulting from chronic microvascular ocular damage.[80,81] The determinants of blood flow to the optic nerve and resulting perfusion pressure are complex and are modified by age (see Chapter 3). There is some evidence that reduction in blood pressure reduces the risk of glaucoma, however, the consistency of this finding is yet to be shown.[67] The relation between diabetes and POAG remains unclear[71] with some studies finding a positive association (with one population-based study finding a doubling of the risk),[82] and other studies finding no association.[83]

Cholesterol and coronary heart disease

Despite hyperlipidaemia being related to cataract, ocular vessel occlusion, and age-related maculo-pathy,[84] case–control studies (based on less than 200 subjects) have shown no difference in serum lipids (total cholesterol, low-density lipoprotein and triglycerides) between glaucomatous and normal patients.[85,86] However, topical β-blockers (used in POAG management) have been reported to lower serum high-density lipoprotein and raise triglyceride levels[87] (mirroring systemic effects of β-blockers);[88,89] these effects are strong risk factors for cardiovascular disease.[90] Hence, it has been proposed that pharmaceutical glaucoma management should be modified in those at higher cardiovascular risk, and that medications that do not adversely effect serum lipids should be preferentially used (e.g. prostaglandin analogues and sympathomimetics).[88] However, the association between chronic use of topical β-blockers and cardiovascular events (such as myocardial infarction, angina, stroke and transient ischaemic attacks) remains to be fully quantified.[91–93] A recent large scale, case–control study (with 667 cases and 6667 controls) showed that subjects using statins and other lipid-lowering medications, especially among those with cardiovascular and lipid diseases, have a lower risk of POAG compared to those not receiving these types of medication.[94] However, further epidemiological studies are needed to establish whether hyperlipidaemic therapy offers any protection against POAG.

Vasospasm

Associations between vasospastic phenomena (cold extremities, migraine, Raynaud's syndrome) and glaucoma have led to an ischaemic hypothesis for glaucoma;[95,96] a hypothesis which has both biological and experimental supporting evidence.[97,98]

However, the relationship between diagnosis of POAG and vasospastic phenomena requires further epidemiological investigation.

Other systemic disorders

There is a suggestion for other emerging associations, such as the relation between Alzheimer's disease (or dementia) and glaucoma.[99–100] However, the putative role of these disorders in relation to glaucoma needs to be replicated in other studies.

1.5 SCREENING

Screening is the systematic application of a test or enquiry to identify individuals at sufficient risk of a disorder to benefit from further investigation or direct preventive action, among persons who have not sought medical attention on account of symptoms of that disorder.

Wald (2004)[1]

Screening is concerned with the detection of a disorder at the asymptomatic stage, i.e. the person is not already receiving any intervention for that disorder. Screening is often carried out to identify a group of individuals at sufficient risk to go on to have a diagnostic test. Cases of POAG identified in patients who choose to attend for an eye examination is not screening per se but identification within a self-selecting group. Whether screening for a particular disorder is worthwhile depends on many factors:[101]

1. The condition being screened for should be an important health problem.
2. The natural history of the condition should be well understood.
3. There should be a detectable early stage.
4. Treatment at an early stage should be of more benefit than at a later stage.
5. There should be a suitable test for the early stage.
6. The test should be acceptable.
7. Intervals for repeating the screening test should be determined.
8. There should be adequate health provision for the extra clinical workload resulting from the screening.
9. The risks of treatment, both physical and psychological, should be less than the benefits.
10. The costs should be balanced against the benefits.

In terms of POAG, items (1), (3) and (6) apply and there is some support for treatment slowing down the progression of visual field defects (4). A systematic review of 114 randomised controlled trials showed that treatment effectively lowers IOP, but only three trials provided data on vision-related outcomes and these did not show a beneficial effect of lowering IOP on visual function.[102] A Cochrane Review of interventions in patients with 'normal tension' glaucoma (glaucoma with IOP in the 'normal range') concluded that IOP lowering had a beneficial effect on visual field outcome only if cataract development was taken into account.[103] However, more recent evidence from a randomised controlled trial, in which a control group did not receive therapy, suggests that 'early' treatment of glaucoma delays progression of the disease.[104] After 6 years of follow-up 62% of the control group and 45% in the treated group had evidence of glaucomatous progression based on visual field or optic disc changes. The relative risk of progression in the treated group vs control group was 0.73 (45% ÷ 62%) i.e. 27% lower in the treated group. Another randomised trial of ocular hypertensives found that the incidence of glaucoma was 60% lower in the treated group compared with the control group.[105]

The Advanced Glaucoma Intervention Study,[106] based on patients with medically uncontrolled glaucoma, reported that worse visual field status at baseline and older age were associated with poorer visual field and visual acuity prognosis after 10 years of follow-up. Other studies have shown that, in general, patients who attend clinics have more advanced glaucoma than those detected by a population survey, in terms of having more advanced visual field loss, higher IOPs, and higher incidence of bilateral disease.[107] Risk factors for more advanced presentation of glaucoma include older age, male sex and those of lower social class. Black Caribbean patients were found to present with more advanced disease than white patients.[60,61] The current belief is that if patients could be treated at an earlier stage of the disease the long-term prognosis for visual function would be improved. The ideal would be to detect the disease before functional loss has occurred, but such an ideal is difficult to achieve. Given that no treatment is without side effects or potential harm, intervention has to be justified by the high probability that worse will ensue if nothing is done. So identification of functional loss prior to causing disability may be a reasonable working framework. How this could be best performed is not clear. There are many different methods for detecting functional visual loss and currently there has not been a systematic review of the current evidence from the different methods.

The performance of a screening (or diagnostic) test is usually quantified in terms of three important measures.

- **Detection rate** (sensitivity): This is the proportion of people *with* the disease with positive test results.
- **False-positive rate** (1–specificity): This is the proportion of people *without* the disease with positive test results.
- **Odds of being affected with the disease given a positive result**: This is the ratio of the number of affected individuals with positive test results to the number of unaffected individuals with positive test results.

The terms detection rate and false-positive rate quantify the proportion (this can also be expressed as a percentage) with positive test results in people affected and unaffected by the disease of interest, respectively; they are synonymous with sensitivity and 1–specificity, respectively, but these terms are often confused. Throughout this section detection rate and false-positive rate are used in preference.

Table 1.4 is a hypothetical example using a screening test with a detection rate of 85% and a false-positive rate of 10% to screen 100 000 people with a prevalence of POAG of 2%.

Detection rate = 1700/2000 = 85%

False-positive rate = 9800/98 000 = 10%

In this example screening 100 000 people would result in 11 500 individuals having a positive screening test result for glaucoma (i.e. screen-positive results) of which only 1700 would actually have POAG.

Table 1.4 Hypothetical results from screening 100 000 people using a screening test that has a detection rate of 85% and a false-positive rate of 10%. Prevalence of POAG is taken to be 2%

Screening test result	Definitive diagnosis		
	With POAG	Without POAG	Total
Positive	1700	9800	11 500
Negative	300	88 200	88 500
Total	2000	98 000	100 000

Odds of being affected given a positive screening result = $1700 : 9800 \approx 10 : 58$

Hence, for every 10 people diagnosed as having POAG, 58 would not have POAG, i.e. about 15% (1700/11500 × 100%) of all the screen positives would have POAG. The reason for the low yield from this screening test is due to a combination of a high false-positive rate and low prevalence of the disease. Screening in populations with high prevalence of POAG may be justified, e.g. screening certain ethnic groups (e.g. black Africans), the elderly or individuals with a family history of glaucoma.

From the evidence presented earlier in this chapter it is clear that measuring IOP alone would be a poor screening test, because there is considerable overlap in IOP levels between those with and without POAG, with about half of those with POAG having IOPs within the 'normal range' at screening. Screening on the basis of IOP alone would be even worse than the example given in Table 1.4, with a detection rate of about 50% and a false-positive rate of about 10% (see also section 1.4.1).

Identifying patients on the basis of structural loss at the optic nerve head alone is also a poor screening tool.[108] If a cut-off of CD ratio ≥0.5 is taken, the detection rate is approximately 50–60%, improving slightly if family history is also taken into consideration, but the false-positive rate is too high, approximately 12%. This means that 12% of the entire unaffected population screened would be referred for definitive diagnosis. At a population level this would be impractical. In a small study of 67 patients with newly diagnosed POAG and 145 non-glaucomatous individuals examined by direct ophthalmoscopy, various features of the optic disc were graded.[109] No single cut-off criterion for any of the optic disc parameters performed well. On combining information from all disc parameters, a detection rate of 81% and a false-positive rate of 10% (similar to the example in Table 1.4) was achieved, and the authors concluded that disc assessment in isolation is inadequate for screening. Tielsch et al[108] found, however, that combining disc parameters with IOP only achieved a detection rate of 61% for a 16% false-positive rate. Additionally including age, race, and family history raised the detection rate to 82% but the false-positive rate also increased to 20%.

In summary, the current evidence suggests screening tests can achieve high detection rates (sensitivity) (approximately 70–80%) but the false positive rates (100–specificity expressed as a percentage) are typically as high as 10–30%.[109–113] This means that about 10–30% of all people tested would be referred for further examination or investigation, which would overwhelm the health services.

In most Western societies, population screening for POAG is probably unjustified because:

■ No satisfactory screening test has been identified that would be suitable for mass screening, whether this constitutes measuring a single marker or collection of different markers.

■ POAG prevalence is generally low, so the yield from screening will also be low. This might be partially tackled by restricting screening to the elderly, e.g. those aged 65 years or more.

■ Further evidence is required to establish whether treatment in the presymptomatic phase provides significant reduction in visual disability or visual impairment in the long term. Evidence suggests that treatment delays the deterioration of visual field by approximately 18 months only.[104]

It has been reported that up to 50% of those requiring long-term follow-up care in hospital eye departments are glaucoma patients. It is also likely that only half of the national caseload in the UK is currently being treated. Thus if an effective screening test was identified for population screening for glaucoma it would increase the burden of long-term management of glaucoma patients and co-management schemes will be required to alleviate this burden. Hence a framework for co-management should be established before population screening for glaucoma becomes a reality. Chapter 13 specifically covers aspects of glaucoma co-management.

References

1. Wald NJ. The Epidemiological Approach: An Introduction to Epidemiology in Medicine. London: Royal Society of Medicine Press; 2004.
2. Coleman AL. Glaucoma. Lancet 1999; 354:1803–1810.
3. Kitazawa Y, Horie T, Aoki S, et al. Untreated ocular hypertension. A long-term prospective study. Arch Ophthalmol 1977; 95:1180–1184.
4. David R, Livingston DG, Luntz MH. Ocular hypertension—a long-term follow-up of treated and untreated patients. Br J Ophthalmol 1977; 61:668–674.
5. Quigley HA, Enger C, Katz J, et al. Risk factors for the development of glaucomatous visual field loss in ocular hypertension. Arch Ophthalmol 1994; 112:644–649.
6. Leske MC, Connell AM, Wu SY, et al. Incidence of open-angle glaucoma: the Barbados Eye Studies. The Barbados Eye Studies Group. Arch Ophthalmol 2001; 119:89–95.
7. Le A, Mukesh BN, McCarty CA, et al. Risk factors associated with the incidence of open-angle glaucoma: the visual impairment project. Invest Ophthalmol Vis Sci 2003; 44:3783–3789.
8. Congdon N, Wang F, Tielsch JM. Issues in the epidemiology and population-based screening of primary angle-closure glaucoma. Surv Ophthalmol 1992; 36:411–423.
9. Bengtsson B. The prevalence of glaucoma. Br J Ophthalmol 1981; 65:46–49.
10. Coffey M, Reidy A, Wormald R, et al. Prevalence of glaucoma in the west of Ireland. Br J Ophthalmol 1993; 77:17–21.
11. Tielsch JM, Sommer A, Witt K, et al. Blindness and visual impairment in an American urban population. The Baltimore Eye Survey. Arch Ophthalmol 1990; 108:286–290.

12. Tielsch JM, Sommer A, Katz J, et al. Racial variations in the prevalence of primary open-angle glaucoma. The Baltimore Eye Survey. JAMA 1991; 266:369–374.

13. Hollows FC, Graham PA. Intra-ocular pressure, glaucoma, and glaucoma suspects in a defined population. Br J Ophthalmol 1966; 50: 570–586.

14. Mason RP, Kosoko O, Wilson MR, et al. National survey of the prevalence and risk factors of glaucoma in St. Lucia, West Indies. Part I. Prevalence findings. Ophthalmology 1989; 96:1363–1368.

15. Leske MC, Connell AM, Schachat AP, et al. The Barbados Eye Study. Prevalence of open angle glaucoma. Arch Ophthalmol 1994; 112:821–829.

16. Wormald RP, Basauri E, Wright LA, et al. The African Caribbean Eye Survey: risk factors for glaucoma in a sample of African Caribbean people living in London. Eye 1994; 8(Pt 3):315–320.

17. Buhrmann RR, Quigley HA, Barron Y, et al. Prevalence of glaucoma in a rural East African population. Invest Ophthalmol Vis Sci 2000; 41:40–48.

18. Rotchford AP, Kirwan JF, Muller MA, et al. Temba glaucoma study: a population-based cross-sectional survey in urban South Africa. Ophthalmology 2003; 110:376–382.

19. Awasthi P, Sarbhai KP, Banerjee SC, et al. Prevalence study of glaucoma in rural areas. Indian J Ophthalmol 1975; 23:1–5.

20. Hu CN. An epidemiologic study of glaucoma in Shunyi County, Beijing. Zhonghua Yan Ke Za Zhi 1989; 25:115–119.

21. Shiose Y, Kitazawa Y, Tsukahara S, et al. Epidemiology of glaucoma in Japan—a nationwide glaucoma survey. Jpn J Ophthalmol 1991; 35:133–155.

22. Foster PJ, Baasanhu J, Alsbirk PH, et al. Glaucoma in Mongolia. A population-based survey in Hovsgol province, northern Mongolia. Arch Ophthalmol 1996; 114:1235–1241.

23. Jacob A, Thomas R, Koshi SP, et al. Prevalence of primary glaucoma in an urban south Indian population. Indian J Ophthalmol 1998; 46:81–86.

24. Foster PJ, Oen FTS, Machin D, et al. The prevalence of glaucoma in Chinese residents of Singapore—A cross-sectional population survey of the Tanjong Pagar District. Arch Ophthalmol 2000; 118:1105–1111.

25. Metheetrairut A, Singalavanija A, Ruangvaravate N, et al. Evaluation of screening tests and prevalence of glaucoma: integrated health research program for the Thai elderly. J Med Assoc Thai 2002; 85:147–153.

26. Ramakrishnan R, Nirmalan PK, Krishnadas R, et al. Glaucoma in a rural population of southern India: the Aravind comprehensive eye survey. Ophthalmology 2003; 110:1484–1490.

27. Iwase A, Suzuki Y, Araie M, et al. The prevalence of primary open-angle glaucoma in Japanese: the Tajimi Study. Ophthalmology 2004; 111:1641–1648.

28. Arkell SM, Lightman DA, Sommer A, et al. The prevalence of glaucoma among Eskimos of northwest Alaska. Arch Ophthalmol 1987; 105:482–485.

29. Bankes JL, Perkins ES, Tsolakis S, et al. Bedford glaucoma survey. Br Med J 1968; 1:791–796.

30. Leibowitz HM, Krueger DE, Maunder LR, et al. The Framingham Eye Study monograph: An ophthalmological and epidemiological study of cataract, glaucoma, diabetic retinopathy, macular degeneration, and visual acuity in a general population of 2631 adults, 1973–1975. Surv Ophthalmol 1980; 24:335–610.

31. Ringvold A, Blika S, Elsas T, et al. The middle-Norway eye-screening study. II. Prevalence of simple and capsular glaucoma. Acta Ophthalmol (Copenhagen) 1991; 69:273–280.

32. Klein BE, Klein R, Sponsel WE, et al. Prevalence of glaucoma. The Beaver Dam Eye Study. Ophthalmology 1992; 99:1499–1504.

33. Salmon JF, Mermoud A, Ivey A, et al. The prevalence of primary angle closure glaucoma and open angle glaucoma in Mamre, Western Cape, South Africa. Arch Ophthalmol 1993; 111:1263–1269.

34. Dielemans I, Vingerling JR, Wolfs RC, et al. The prevalence of primary open-angle glaucoma in a population-based study in The Netherlands. The Rotterdam Study. Ophthalmology 1994; 101:1851–1855.

35. Giuffre G, Giammanco R, Dardanoni G, et al. Prevalence of glaucoma and distribution of intraocular pressure in a population. The Casteldaccia Eye Study. Acta Ophthalmol Scand 1995; 73:222–225.

36. Hirvela H, Tuulonen A, Laatikainen L. Intraocular pressure and prevalence of glaucoma in elderly people in Finland: a population-based study. Int Ophthalmol 1994; 18:299–307.

37. Mitchell P, Smith W, Attebo K, et al. Prevalence of open-angle glaucoma in Australia. The Blue

Mountains Eye Study. Ophthalmology 1996; 103:1661–1669.

38. Cedrone C, Culasso F, Cesareo M, et al. Prevalence of glaucoma in Ponza, Italy: a comparison with other studies. Ophthalmic Epidemiol 1997; 4:59–72.

39. Wensor MD, McCarty CA, Stanislavsky YL, et al. The prevalence of glaucoma in the Melbourne Visual Impairment Project. Ophthalmology 1998; 105:733–739.

40. Bonomi L, Marchini G, Marraffa M, et al. Prevalence of glaucoma and intraocular pressure distribution in a defined population. The Egna-Neumarkt Study. Ophthalmology 1998; 105:209–215.

41. Reidy A, Minassian DC, Vafidis G, et al. Prevalence of serious eye disease and visual impairment in a north London population: population based, cross sectional study. BMJ 1998; 316:1643–1646.

42. Quigley HA, West SK, Rodriguez J, et al. The prevalence of glaucoma in a population-based study of Hispanic subjects: Proyecto VER. Arch Ophthalmol 2001; 119:1819–1826.

43. Mann I, Potter D. Geographic ophthalmology. A preliminary study of the Maoris of New Zealand. Am J Ophthalmol 1969; 67:358–369.

44. Taylor HR. Prevalence and causes of blindness in Australian aborigines. Med J Aust 1980; 1:71–76.

45. Rudnicka AR, Mt-Isa S, Owen CG, et al. Variations in primary open angle glaucoma prevalence by age, gender and race: a Bayesian meta-analysis. Invest Ophthalmol Vis Sci 2006; 47:4254–4261.

46. Bengtsson BO. Incidence of manifest glaucoma. Br J Ophthalmol 1989; 73:483–487.

47. Dreyer EB, Lipton SA. New perspectives on glaucoma. JAMA 1999; 281:306–308.

48. Sommer A, Tielsch JM, Katz J, et al. Relationship between intraocular pressure and primary open angle glaucoma among white and black Americans. The Baltimore Eye Survey. Arch Ophthalmol 1991; 109:1090–1095.

49. Klein BE, Klein R, Linton KL. Intraocular pressure in an American community. The Beaver Dam Eye Study. Invest Ophthalmol Vis Sci 1992; 33:2224–2228.

50. Bonomi L, Marchini G, Marraffa M, et al. Vascular risk factors for primary open angle glaucoma: the Egna-Neumarkt Study. Ophthalmology 2000; 107:1287–1293.

51. Mitchell P, Hourihan F, Sandbach J, et al. The relationship between glaucoma and myopia: the Blue Mountains Eye Study. Ophthalmology 1999; 106:2010–2015.

52. Wong TY, Klein BE, Klein R, et al. Refractive errors, intraocular pressure, and glaucoma in a white population. Ophthalmology 2003; 110:211–217.

53. Grodum K, Heijl A, Bengtsson B. Refractive error and glaucoma. Acta Ophthalmol Scand 2001; 79:560–566.

54. Wu SY, Nemesure B, Leske MC. Refractive errors in a black adult population: the Barbados Eye Study. Invest Ophthalmol Vis Sci 1999; 40:2179–2184.

55. Leske MC, Nemesure B, He Q, et al. Patterns of open-angle glaucoma in the Barbados Family Study. Ophthalmology 2001; 108:1015–1022.

56. Schoff EO, Hattenhauer MG, Ing HH, et al. Estimated incidence of open-angle glaucoma in Olmsted County, Minnesota. Ophthalmology 2001; 108:882–886.

57. Mukesh BN, McCarty CA, Rait JL, et al. Five-year incidence of open-angle glaucoma: the visual impairment project. Ophthalmology 2002; 109:1047–1051.

58. Owen CG, Carey IM, De Wilde S, et al. The epidemiology of medical treatment for glaucoma and ocular hypertension in the United Kingdom: 1994 to 2003. Br J Ophthalmol 2006; 90:861–868.

59. Wormald R, Fraser S, Bunce C. Time to look again at sight tests. BMJ 1997; 314:245.

60. Fraser S, Bunce C, Wormald R, et al. Deprivation and late presentation of glaucoma: case-control study. BMJ 2001; 322:639–643.

61. Fraser S, Bunce C, Wormald R. Retrospective analysis of risk factors for late presentation of chronic glaucoma. Br J Ophthalmol 1999; 83:24–28.

62. Tielsch JM, Sommer A, Katz J, et al. Socioeconomic status and visual impairment among urban Americans. Baltimore Eye Survey Research Group. Arch Ophthalmol 1991; 109:637–641.

63. Klein BE, Klein R, Ritter LL. Relationship of drinking alcohol and smoking to prevalence of open-angle glaucoma. The Beaver Dam Eye Study. Ophthalmology 1993; 100:1609–1613.

64. Bonovas S, Filioussi K, Tsantes A, et al. Epidemiological association between cigarette smoking and primary open-angle glaucoma: a meta-analysis. Public Health 2004; 118:256–261.

65. Gottfredsdottir MS, Sverrisson T, Musch DC, et al. Chronic open-angle glaucoma and associated ophthalmic findings in monozygotic twins and their spouses in Iceland. J Glaucoma 1999; 8:134–139.

66. Mitchell P, Rochtchina E, Lee AJ, et al. Bias in self-reported family history and relationship to glaucoma: the Blue Mountains Eye Study. Ophthalmic Epidemiol 2002; 9:333–345.

67. Weih LM, Mukesh BN, McCarty CA, et al. Association of demographic, familial, medical, and ocular factors with intraocular pressure. Arch Ophthalmol 2001; 119:875–880.

68. Nemesure B, Leske MC, He Q, et al. Analyses of reported family history of glaucoma: a preliminary investigation. The Barbados Eye Study Group. Ophthalmic Epidemiol 1996; 3:135–141.

69. Tielsch JM, Katz J, Sommer A, et al. Family history and risk of primary open angle glaucoma. The Baltimore Eye Survey. Arch Ophthalmol 1994; 112:69–73.

70. Wolfs RC, Klaver CC, Ramrattan RS, et al. Genetic risk of primary open-angle glaucoma. Population-based familial aggregation study. Arch Ophthalmol 1998; 116:1640–1645.

71. Quigley HA. Open-angle glaucoma. N Engl J Med 1993; 328:1097–1106.

72. Weisschuh N, Schiefer U. Progress in the genetics of glaucoma. Dev Ophthalmol 2003; 37:83–93.

73. Challa P. Glaucoma genetics: advancing new understandings of glaucoma pathogenesis. Int Ophthalmol Clin 2004; 44:167–185.

74. Cohen CS, Allingham RR. The dawn of genetic testing for glaucoma. Curr Opin Ophthalmol 2004; 15:75–79.

75. Morgan RW, Drance SM. Chronic open-angle glaucoma and ocular hypertension. An epidemiological study. Br J Ophthalmol 1975; 59:211–215.

76. Leske MC, Podgor MJ. Intraocular pressure, cardiovascular risk variables, and visual field defects. Am J Epidemiol 1983; 118:280–287.

77. Wilson MR, Hertzmark E, Walker AM, et al. A case-control study of risk factors in open angle glaucoma. Arch Ophthalmol 1987; 105:1066–1071.

78. Dielemans I, Vingerling JR, Algra D, et al. Primary open-angle glaucoma, intraocular pressure, and systemic blood pressure in the general elderly population. The Rotterdam Study. Ophthalmology 1995; 102:54–60.

79. Tielsch JM, Katz J, Sommer A, et al. Hypertension, perfusion pressure, and primary open-angle glaucoma. A population-based assessment. Arch Ophthalmol 1995; 113:216–221.

80. Graham S. Are vascular factors involved in glaucomatous damage? Aust N Z J Ophthalmol 1999; 27:354–356.

81. Laatikainen L. Fluorescein angiographic studies of the peripapillary and perilimbal regions in simple, capsular and low-tension glaucoma. Acta Ophthalmol Suppl 1971; 111:3–83.

82. Mitchell P, Smith W, Chey T, et al. Open-angle glaucoma and diabetes: the Blue Mountains eye study, Australia. Ophthalmology 1997; 104:712–718.

83. Tielsch JM, Katz J, Quigley HA, et al. Diabetes, intraocular pressure, and primary open-angle glaucoma in the Baltimore Eye Survey. Ophthalmology 1995; 102:48–53.

84. Flammer J, Haefliger IO, Orgul S, et al. Vascular dysregulation: a principal risk factor for glaucomatous damage? J Glaucoma 1999; 8:212–219.

85. Goldberg I, Hollows FC, Kass MA, et al. Systemic factors in patients with low-tension glaucoma. Br J Ophthalmol 1981; 65:56–62.

86. Chisholm IA, Stead S. Plasma lipid patterns in patients with suspected glaucoma. Can J Ophthalmol 1988; 23:164–167.

87. Goldberg I. Should beta blockers be abandoned as initial monotherapy in chronic open angle glaucoma? The controversy. Br J Ophthalmol 2002; 86:691–692.

88. Stewart WC, Osterman J. Serum lipid physiology and the influence of glaucoma medications. Surv Ophthalmol 1998; 43:233–244.

89. Mitchell P, Wang JJ, Cumming RG, et al. Long-term topical timolol and blood lipids: the Blue Mountains Eye Study. J Glaucoma 2000; 9:174–178.

90. Pocock SJ, Shaper AG, Phillips AN. Concentrations of high density lipoprotein cholesterol, triglycerides, and total cholesterol in ischaemic heart disease. BMJ 1989; 298:998–1002.

91. Armaly MF. Glaucoma. Arch Ophthalmol 1972; 88:439–460.

92. Drance SM. Some factors in the production of low tension glaucoma. Br J Ophthalmol 1972; 56:229–242.

93. Klein BE, Klein R. Intraocular pressure and cardiovascular risk variables. Arch Ophthalmol 1981; 99:837–839.

94. McGwin G Jr, McNeal S, Owsley C, et al. Statins and other cholesterol-lowering medications and the presence of glaucoma. Arch Ophthalmol 2004; 122:822–826.

95. Schulzer M, Drance SM, Carter CJ, et al. Biostatistical evidence for two distinct chronic open angle glaucoma populations. Br J Ophthalmol 1990; 74:196–200.

96. Wang L, Cioffi GA, Van Buskirk EM. The vascular pattern of the optic nerve and its potential relevance in glaucoma. Curr Opin Ophthalmol 1998; 9:24–29.

97. Orgul S, Cioffi GA, Wilson DJ, et al. An endothelin-1 induced model of optic nerve ischemia in the rabbit. Invest Ophthalmol Vis Sci 1996; 37:1860–1869.

98. O'Brien C. Vasospasm and glaucoma. Br J Ophthalmol 1998; 82:855–856.

99. Bayer AU, Keller ON, Ferrari F, et al. Association of glaucoma with neurodegenerative diseases with apoptotic cell death: Alzheimer's disease and Parkinson's disease. Am J Ophthalmol 2002; 133:135–137.

100. Bayer AU, Ferrari F, Erb C. High occurrence rate of glaucoma among patients with Alzheimer's disease. Eur Neurol 2002; 47:165–168.

101. Wilson JM, Jungner YG. Principles of mass screening for disease. Bol Oficina Sanit Panam 1968; 64:281–293.

102. Rossetti L, Marchetti N, Orzalsei N, et al. Randomized clinical trials on medical treatment of glaucoma. Are they appropriate to guide clinical practice? Arch Ophthalmol 1993; 111:96–103.

103. Sycha T, Vass C, Findl O, et al. Interventions for normal tension glaucoma. Cochrane Database Syst Rev 2003:CD002222.

104. Heijl A, Leske MC, Bengtsson B, et al. Reduction of intraocular pressure and glaucoma progression: results from the Early Manifest Glaucoma Trial. Arch Ophthalmol 2002; 120:1268–1279.

105. Kass MA, Heuer DK, Higginbotham EJ, et al. The Ocular Hypertension Treatment Study: a randomized trial determines that topical ocular hypotensive medication delays or prevents the onset of primary open-angle glaucoma. Arch Ophthalmol 2002; 120:701–713.

106. The Advanced Glaucoma Intervention Study (AGIS): 12. Baseline risk factors for sustained loss of visual field and visual acuity in patients with advanced glaucoma. Am J Ophthalmol 2002; 134:499–512.

107. Grodum K, Heijl A, Bengtsson B. A comparison of glaucoma patients identified through mass screening and in routine clinical practice. Acta Ophthalmol Scand 2002; 80:627–631.

108. Tielsch JM, Katz J, Singh K, et al. A population-based evaluation of glaucoma screening: the Baltimore Eye Survey. Am J Epidemiol 1991; 134:1102–1110.

109. Harper R, Reeves B. The sensitivity and specificity of direct ophthalmoscopic optic disc assessment in screening for glaucoma: a multivariate analysis. Graefes Arch Clin Exp Ophthalmol 2000; 238:949–955.

110. Vitale S, Smith TD, Quigley T, et al. Screening performance of functional and structural measurements of neural damage in open-angle glaucoma: a case-control study from the Baltimore Eye Survey. J Glaucoma 2000; 9:346–356.

111. Allen CS, Sponsel WE, Trigo Y, et al. Comparison of the frequency doubling technology screening algorithm and the Humphrey 24–2 SITA-FAST in a large eye screening. Clin Experiment Ophthalmol 2002; 30:8–14.

112. Kothy P, Vargha P, Hollo G. Glaucoma-screening with the Heidelberg Retina Tomograph II. Klin Monatsbl Augenheilkd 2003; 220:540–544.

113. Kalaboukhova L, Lindblom B. Frequency doubling technology and high-pass resolution perimetry in glaucoma and ocular hypertension. Acta Ophthalmol Scand 2003; 81:247–252.

Chapter 2

Production and drainage of aqueous humour

John G Lawrenson

2.1 INTRODUCTION

Knowledge of the production and drainage of aqueous humour is essential for a full understanding of the medical and surgical management of glaucoma. This chapter will outline the composition, dynamics and function of aqueous humour, and describe the role of the ciliary epithelium in aqueous production. Both conventional (i.e. via the canal of Schlemm) and alternative (i.e. uveoscleral) pathways for aqueous outflow will be described in detail. Physiological and pharmacological modulation of aqueous production and drainage will also be reviewed.

2.2 AQUEOUS HUMOUR

Aqueous humour is a transparent colourless fluid that is essential for the nutrition of the avascular cornea and lens, and the removal of metabolic waste products. It also generates an intraocular pressure (IOP) that is determined by the balance between aqueous production and drainage. Although the rate of aqueous production cannot be measured directly in humans, it can be assumed to be proportional to the flow of aqueous through the anterior chamber. Typically this is determined by introducing fluorescein into the eye and measuring its rate of clearance.[1] Flow rates vary between $2\,\mu l/min$ and $3\,\mu l/min$. Much higher flow rates have been recorded during waking hours than during sleep, possibly the result of circadian variation in endogenous hormones. Flow rates also vary with age, showing a 25% decline from 10 to 80 years.[1]

The composition of the aqueous reflects the secretory activity of the ciliary epithelium and the metabolic processes within the eye. The electrolyte concentration is broadly similar to plasma, although the two fluids differ in the concentration of particular electrolytes e.g. Ca^{2+}, Mg^{2+} and HCO_3^-. Aqueous also differs in the concentration of certain organic solutes, e.g. the levels of ascorbate and lactate are much higher than in plasma.[2] In the interests of optical clarity, the aqueous contains a very low concentration of protein that is generally <1% of the level in plasma.[3] This situation is maintained by the blood–aqueous barrier, which acts as an exclusion filter. Inflammation of the anterior uvea can cause a breakdown of this barrier and results in increased levels of protein in the aqueous. The resulting light scatter by protein molecules is manifest clinically as 'flare'.

2.3 THE ANTERIOR CHAMBER AND AQUEOUS DYNAMICS

The anterior chamber is bounded on its front surface by the cornea, and its posterior boundary is formed by the iris and lens. The anterior chamber varies in diameter from 11.3 mm to 12.4 mm. Its depth is greatest axially, and becomes progressively shallower peripherally.[4] Chamber depth is variable (2.9–3.8 mm), being generally greater in myopic eyes and shallower in hyperopes. It also reduces with age (0.1 mm per decade), presumably due to the increased axial width of the lens. Variation in anterior chamber depth also influences the angle formed between the posterior aspect of the corneoscleral limbus and the iris. This angle is significant, since its recess contains the tissues responsible for aqueous drainage. For this reason it is frequently referred to as the 'drainage angle'. It is essential that access to the angle tissues is unimpeded, and anatomical variation in the anterior chamber angle depth can lead to a narrowing of the drainage angle and a predisposition to closed angle glaucoma.

Aqueous is secreted into the posterior chamber by the ciliary epithelium. It passes around the

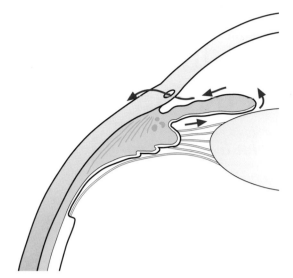

Fig. 2.1 Schematic representation of aqueous dynamics. Arrows indicate the direction of aqueous flow.

equator of the lens, and then flows through the pupil into the anterior chamber (Fig. 2.1). Aqueous circulates within the anterior chamber due to convection currents, which derive from temperature differences between the cornea and iris.[3] Aqueous then leaves the eye via two alternative routes:

- Conventional pathway: through the trabecular meshwork into the canal of Schlemm from where it drains into episcleral veins.
- Uveoscleral pathway: through the ciliary muscle into the supraciliary and suprachoroidal spaces.

Although the trabecular route accounts for the vast majority of aqueous outflow, the development of prostaglandin analogues for the treatment of glaucoma has renewed interest in the uveoscleral pathway.[5] By increasing the proportion of aqueous leaving by this route these agents have proved to be effective ocular hypotensive drugs.[6]

2.4 AQUEOUS PRODUCTION

The raw materials for aqueous humour derive from the highly permeable fenestrated capillaries that supply the ciliary processes of the ciliary body. The major component of aqueous is water that enters the posterior chamber along an osmotic gradient

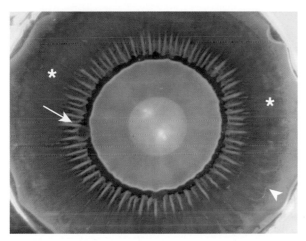

Fig. 2.2 Gross view of the inner surface of the ciliary body. Note the radially orientated ciliary processes of the pars plicata (arrow). The pars plana (asterisk) is featureless and uniformly pigmented. The ora serrata (arrow head) marks the posterior aspect of the ciliary body.

derived from the metabolically driven transport of ions within the ciliary epithelium.[7,8]

2.4.1 ANATOMY OF THE CILIARY BODY

The ciliary body represents the middle part of the uveal tract that extends from the scleral spur to the ora serrata. It can be divided into two anatomical regions (Fig. 2.2):

■ Pars plicata: represents the anterior one-third of the ciliary body, and is characterised by 70–80 radially orientated ridges, which project into the posterior chamber. These ridges are termed ciliary processes, and represent the primary site of aqueous formation.
■ Pars plana: represents the posterior two-thirds of the ciliary body. It is characterised by a smooth and uniformly pigmented surface.

Histologically, the ciliary processes consist of a core of loose connective tissue that contain numerous fenestrated capillaries (Fig. 2.3). The overlying epithelium is a double layer of cuboidal cells. The inner layer, which lies adjacent to the posterior chamber, is non-pigmented, and the outer layer (adjacent to the stroma) is pigmented. Uniquely,

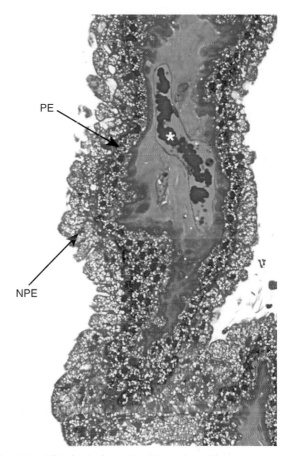

Fig. 2.3 Histological section through a ciliary process. A fibrovascular core (asterisk) is bounded by a double epithelial layer. NPE, non-pigmented epithelium; PE, pigmented epithelium.

ciliary epithelial cells face each other apex to apex, as a result of the invagination of the optic cup during the embryological development of the eye. The pigmented epithelium (PE) is continuous with the retinal pigment epithelium and contains numerous round or elliptical pigment granules (melanosomes) (Fig. 2.4). The basal surface of these cells is highly convoluted, to facilitate solute uptake from the stroma. Moreover, numerous gap junctions occur between PE and non-pigmented epithelial cells (NPE) to allow the intercellular exchange of ions and metabolites. The NPE, which is the forward continuation of the neuroretina, contains large numbers of mitochondria and a pronounced endoplasmic reticulum. As with the PE, the NPE displays a convoluted basal membrane to

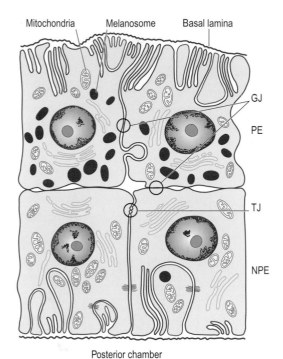

Fig. 2.4 Diagrammatic representation of the ultrastructure of the ciliary epithelium. NPE, non-pigmented epithelium; PE, pigmented epithelium; GJ, gap junction; TJ, tight junction.

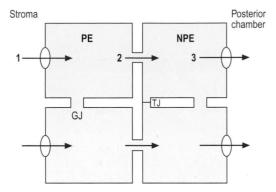

Fig. 2.5 Schematic representation of the steps involved in aqueous production in the ciliary epithelium. 1. The uptake of plasma-derived ions from the ciliary stroma across the basolateral surface of the pigmented epithelium (PE). 2. The movement of ions from PE into non-pigmented epithelium (NPE) via gap junctions (GJ). 3. The active transport of ions from the NPE into the posterior chamber. TJ, tight junction.

increase the surface area across which ions can be transported. Tight junctions are found between adjacent NPE cells. These junctions are the primary site of the blood–aqueous barrier, and also maintain the transepithelial potential difference across the ciliary epithelium.[7]

2.4.2 MECHANISM OF AQUEOUS PRODUCTION

Over the years several theories have been proposed for aqueous production including: simple diffusion, ultrafiltration and active secretion.[9] It is now widely recognised that the active secretion of ions across the ciliary epithelium is the primary mechanism for the formation of aqueous. This creates an osmotic gradient that allows the passive flow of water into the posterior chamber. The precise details of the ion transport mechanisms involved have not been fully elucidated, however it is accepted that the process involves three sequential steps (Fig. 2.5):

1. The uptake of plasma-derived ions from the ciliary stroma across the basolateral surface of the PE.
2. The movement of ions from PE into NPE via gap junctions.
3. The active transport of ions from the NPE into the posterior chamber.

Ions are transported via distinct transporter proteins (Fig. 2.6) and several ionic species are known to be actively secreted by the ciliary epithelium (Fig. 2.7). Sodium and chloride is taken up into PE cells from the stroma via Na^+/H^+ and Cl^-/HCO_3^- antiports and the Na^+-K^+-$2Cl^-$ symport.[8] NPE cells release Na^+ and Cl^- into the aqueous humour via the Na^+K^+ ATPase transporter and chloride channels, respectively. The involvement of Na^+K^+ ATPase in aqueous formation has been known for many years, and this transporter has been histochemically localised to the ciliary epithelium in a variety of species.[10] Inhibition of Na^+ K^+ ATPase with the glycoside ouabain leads to a 30–50% reduction in secretion.[11] The role of HCO_3^- in aqueous formation is also well established. Carbonic anhydrase (CA), an enzyme that leads to HCO_3^- formation via the reversible hydration of carbon dioxide, seems to play a critical role. Although the human ciliary epithelium does not show a net transepithelial transport of HCO_3^-, the

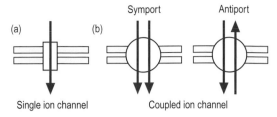

Fig. 2.6 Classification of membrane ion transporters. (a) Single ion channel. (b) Two types of coupled ion transporter. A symport moves ions across the plasma membrane in the same direction and an antiport moves ions in opposite directions.

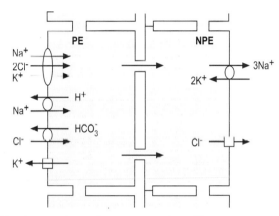

Fig. 2.7 Schematic representation of ion transport pathways involved in aqueous production.

movement of HCO_3^- is coupled to the flux of Cl^-. It has been suggested that the IOP lowering effects of carbonic anhydrase inhibitors such as acetazolamide are likely to be due to an indirect effect on Cl^- transport.[12]

2.4.3 REGULATION OF AQUEOUS SECRETION

Physiological

Aqueous secretion is precisely regulated, principally through the action of the β-adrenergic system. Receptors of the β-2 subtype predominate in the ciliary processes.[13] These receptors are positively coupled, via intermediate G-proteins, to the enzyme complex adenylate cyclase that catalyses

the conversion of ATP into the second messenger cAMP. Elevated cAMP activates protein kinase A, which in turn regulates ion transport and therefore aqueous secretion.[9] In particular, cAMP has been shown to play a crucial role in the modulation of Cl^- transport.[14] Another possible regulatory mechanism for aqueous secretion is via adenosine (derived from ATP) which binds to specific adenosine receptors that in turn modulate ion transport.[15]

Pharmacological

Identification of the precise mechanism by which IOP-lowering drugs exert their effect is difficult to determine. Possible mechanisms include: increased outflow facility, reduced ciliary blood flow, as well as a direct effect on aqueous secretion. β-antagonists (e.g. timolol) or α-agonists (e.g. clonidine) have both been shown to reduce aqueous secretion. Substantial reductions in aqueous secretion have also been demonstrated with carbonic anhydrase inhibitors (e.g. dorzolamide).

2.5 AQUEOUS DRAINAGE

In 1921, Siedel provided the first convincing evidence for the existence of a pathway for aqueous outflow.[16] Following the introduction of a dye into the anterior chamber, episcleral vessels on the surface of the eye became coloured, establishing a potential drainage route into the venous system. Later definitive confirmation of an aqueous outflow pathway was provided by the description of aqueous veins, and the subsequent confirmation of their connectivity with the canal of Schlemm.[17,18]

2.5.1 CONVENTIONAL DRAINAGE PATHWAY

The conventional outflow pathway represents the primary route by which aqueous leaves the eye (Fig. 2.8), passing sequentially through the trabecular meshwork and canal of Schlemm, from where a series of direct (aqueous veins) or indirect (collector channels) pathways drain the aqueous into the venous system at the ocular surface.[19]

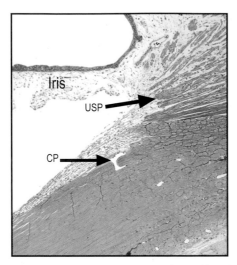

Fig. 2.8 Histological section through the filtration angle showing aqueous outflow pathways. CP, conventional pathway through the canal of Schlemm; USP, uveoscleral pathway.

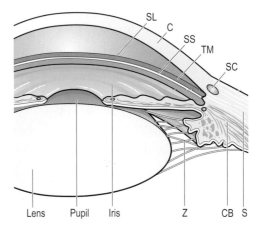

Fig. 2.9 Diagrammatic representation of the gonioscopic appearance of the angle tissues. SL, Schwalbe's line; SS, scleral spur; TM, trabecular meshwork; C, cornea; SC, Schlemm's canal; Z, zonules; CB, ciliary body; S, sclera.

Gross anatomy

The external features of the pathway can be visualised gonioscopically. Schwalbe's line is the most anterior structure, and represents the termination of Descemet's membrane and the transition from corneal endothelium to trabecular cells. In the absence of pigment, the trabecular meshwork appears as a featureless band, approximately 750 µm in width. The posterior border of the trabecular meshwork is marked by a pale translucent ridge that corresponds to the location of the scleral spur (Fig. 2.9).

Microscopic anatomy

In meridional section the trabecular meshwork and canal of Schlemm can be seen to lie within a scleral sulcus that encircles the anterior chamber angle. The trabecular meshwork (TM) is triangular in profile, with its base opposite the scleral spur and its apex adjacent to Schwalbe's line (Fig. 2.10). Anatomically, the meshwork can be resolved into three distinct regions[20] (Fig. 2.11):

- Uveal meshwork
- Corneoscleral meshwork
- Juxta-canalicular tissue (cribriform layer).

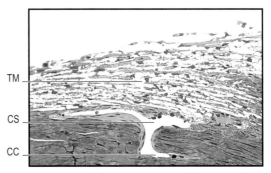

Fig. 2.10 Histological section through trabecular meshwork and canal of Schlemm. TM, trabecular meshwork; CS, canal of Schlemm; CC, collector channel.

The uveal meshwork makes up the inner part of the TM and consists of an irregular net-like structure, formed from one to three layers of cord-like trabeculae that stretch from the iris root to the peripheral cornea. This arrangement creates large intertrabecular spaces ranging from 25 µm to 75 µm in diameter. The corneoscleral meshwork consists of 8–15 layers of flattened sheets extending from the scleral spur to the anterior border of the scleral sulcus. Perforations within the trabecular sheets allow aqueous to percolate through to the endothelial meshwork that lies adjacent to the canal of Schlemm. This juxtacanalicular tissue

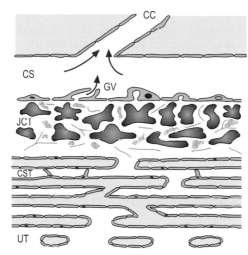

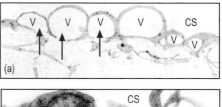

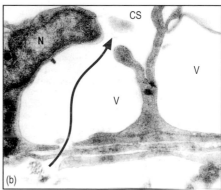

Fig. 2.11 Diagrammatic representation of the trabecular meshwork. UT, uveal trabeculae; CST, corneoscleral trabeculae; JCT, juxtacanalicular tissue; CS, canal of Schlemm; CC, collector channel; GV, giant vacuole.

Fig. 2.12 (a) Electron micrograph of the inner wall of the canal of Schlemm (CS) showing numerous giant vacuoles (V). (b) Detail of a giant vacuole showing apical and basal openings forming a patent transendothelial pathway from the trabecular meshwork into the canal of Schlemm.

(JCT) consists of dendritic endothelial cells linked by gap junctions. The space between cells is composed of plaques of collagen and elastic-like material embedded in a proteoglycan matrix. The JCT represents the main site of the resistance within the outflow system, and is essential for the generation of an IOP.[21] In addition to providing resistance to outflow, the TM also acts as a filter, and trabecular cells have a selective phagocytic capacity. Under normal circumstances the TM can effectively filter and destroy particulate matter, e.g. pigment and the breakdown products of blood. However, overloading may contribute to the pathogenesis of various forms of obstructive secondary glaucoma.[22]

Canal of Schlemm

The canal of Schlemm is a circular venous channel approximately 36 mm in circumference that lies deep within the scleral sulcus. It is elliptical in cross section, although it occasionally splits to form a double lumen. The walls of the canal are made up of a single layer of spindle-shaped endothelial cells that are elongated in the long axis of the canal. The structure and function of the inner wall has received a great deal of attention, since it is the site

that regulates aqueous entry from the TM. Inner wall cells are linked together by tight junctions. At low IOPs these junctions allow only small amounts of aqueous to pass between cells, however it is likely that permeability through this pathway increases with increased IOP.[23] A characteristic feature of the inner wall is the presence of large invaginations termed 'giant vacuoles'. The number and size of these vacuoles increases with IOP,[24] suggesting a potential role in the regulation of aqueous outflow. Electron microscopy reveals that many of these vacuoles show basal and apical openings, forming transcellular pores to allow the passage of aqueous (Fig. 2.12). Transcellular pores, however, are not purely limited to vacuoles.[23]

From the canal of Schlemm, collector channels deliver aqueous into the intrascleral venous plexus that connects with episcleral veins (Fig. 2.13). Aqueous veins represent a special case where mixing of aqueous with blood occurs at the ocular surface. Aqueous veins were first described by Ascher in 1942,[17] and were one of the earliest

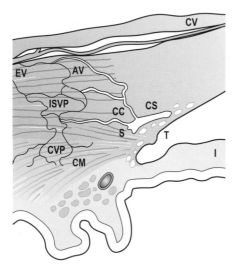

Fig. 2.13 Schematic representation showing the pathways from the canal of Schlemm to the surface of the eye. CS, canal of Schlemm; CC, collector channel; S, scleral spur; T, trabecular meshwork; CM, ciliary muscle; CVP, ciliary venous plexus; ISVP, intrascleral venous plexus; EV, episcleral vein; AV, aqueous vein; CV, conjunctival vessel; I, iris.

demonstrations of aqueous circulation. Where aqueous veins meet episcleral vessels blood and aqueous do not immediately mix and laminar flow is visible. The pressure within the drainage system decreases from the anterior chamber through to the ocular surface. Consequently aqueous flows down a pressure gradient.

2.5.2 REGULATION OF AQUEOUS OUTFLOW

Recent studies have shown that trabecular cells have smooth-muscle-like contractile properties.[20,25] It is possible therefore that trabecular contraction and relaxation may influence outflow. It has been suggested that the trabecular meshwork and ciliary muscle act as functional antagonists, and total outflow is determined by the contractility balance between the ciliary muscle and trabecular meshwork.[25] Ciliary muscle contraction widens the pores within the trabecular meshwork and increases the facility for outflow, whereas trabecular contraction reduces outflow.

The overall effect of various anti-glaucoma drugs on outflow (and thus IOP) is a function of their influence on the trabecular meshwork and the ciliary muscle. For example, the IOP-lowering effect of pilocarpine is due to its more pronounced effect on ciliary muscle contraction.[26]

2.5.3 ALTERNATIVE OUTFLOW ROUTE: UVEOSCLERAL PATHWAY

This alternative outflow pathway was first described by Bill in the 1960s,[27] and has recently attracted renewed attention.[5] Since there is no epithelial barrier between the anterior chamber and the ciliary body, aqueous is able to enter the loose connective tissue in front of the ciliary muscle and pass between the muscle fibres into the supraciliary and suprachoroidal spaces (see Fig. 2.8). From here it can potentially be absorbed by vessels draining the uvea. In contrast with the conventional outflow pathway, uveoscleral outflow is not pressure dependent and its contribution to aqueous outflow is thus the same in eyes with low and high IOP. Direct measurements of aged cadaver eyes estimate that up to 15% of outflow is via this route although more recent indirect evidence in younger eyes has suggested much higher values.[5] The pathway can be modulated pharmacologically. Pilocarpine decreases outflow by this route whereas adrenaline increases it (via a relaxation of the ciliary muscle). The pressure-lowering action of prostaglandin analogues, e.g. latanoprost, is thought to be the result of an increase in uveoscleral outflow. These drugs stimulate the prostaglandin $F_{2\alpha}$ receptor which in turn activates the regulatory protein c-fos to produce matrix metalloproteinase enzymes. These enzymes break down collagen within the extracellular matrix leading to a remodelling of the uveoscleral pathway.[6]

2.5.4 AQUEOUS OUTFLOW PATHWAYS IN GLAUCOMA

The effects of various pathological processes on aqueous outflow pathways are well documented.[20,22] A variety of secondary glaucomas can arise from the obstruction of the intertrabecular spaces by cellular or non-cellular material including: inflammatory cell infiltration, red cells, pigment, lens debris and exfoliation material. In susceptible individuals corticosteroids can also cause elevation of IOP and glaucoma. The pathogenic mechanism in such cases seems to be an increased outflow resistance caused by an accumulation of a basement membrane-like material adjacent to the canal of Schlemm.[20] In contrast, the pathogenesis of primary open angle glaucoma remains elusive. A fundamental problem is the inability to differentiate between the changes seen as part of the normal ageing process and those seen in glaucoma.[22] However, one structural difference that seems to correlate with the severity of glaucoma is the presence of 'plaque-like' deposits in the juxtacanalicular layer.[20] The significance of these changes is currently unclear, however the application of molecular biology techniques to the study of trabecular cells and their pathological response to a variety of stimuli may in the future provide the necessary insights.

References

1. Brubaker RF. Flow of aqueous in humans. Invest Ophthalmol Vis Sci 1991; 32:3145–3166.
2. Davson H. The intra-ocular fluids. In: Davson H, ed. The Eye. New York: Academic Press; 1969.
3. Freddo TF. Shifting the paradigm of the blood-aqueous barrier. Exp Eye Res 2001; 73:581–592.
4. Duke-Elder S, Wybar KC. System of Ophthalmology. Vol. II. The Anatomy of the Visual System. London: Kimpton; 1961.
5. Alm A. Uveoscleral outflow. Eye 2000; 14:488–491.
6. Crowston JG, Weinreb RN. Glaucoma medication and aqueous humour dynamics. Curr Opin Ophthalmol 2005; 16:94–100.
7. To CH, Kong CW, Chan CY, et al. The mechanism of aqueous humour formation. Clin Exp Optom 2002; 85:335–349.
8. Civan MM, Macknight ADC. The ins and outs of aqueous humour secretion. Exp Eye Res 2004; 78:625–631.
9. Sears ML. Formation of aqueous humour. In: Albert DM, Jakobiec FA, eds. Principles and Practice of Ophthalmology. Philadelphia: WB Saunders; 1994.
10. Cole DF. The secretion of aqueous humour. Exp Eye Res Suppl 1977; 25:161–176.
11. Maren TH. Ion secretion into the posterior aqueous humour of dogs and monkeys. Exp Eye Res Suppl 1977; 25:245–247.
12. To CH, Do CW, Zamudio AC, et al. Model of ionic transport for bovine ciliary epithelium: effect of acetazolamide and HCO_3^-. Am J Physiol Cell Physiol 2001; 280:C1521–1530.
13. Wax MB, Molinoff PB. Distribution and properties of beta-adrenergic receptors in human iris-ciliary body. Invest Ophthalmol Vis Sci 1987; 28:420–430.
14. Do CW, Kong CW, To CH. cAMP inhibits transepithelial chloride secretion across bovine ciliary body/epithelium. Invest Ophthalmol Vis Sci 2004; 45:3638–3643.
15. Civan MM. The fall and rise of active chloride transport: implications for regulation of intraocular pressure. J Exp Zoolog A Comp Exp Biol 2003; 300:5–13.
16. Siedel E. Uber der Abfluss des Kammerwassers aus der vorderen Augenkammer. Graefes Arch Clin Exp Ophthalmol 1921; 104:357–402.
17. Ascher KW. Aqueous veins. Preliminary note. Am J Ophthalmol 1942; 25:31–38.
18. Ashton N. Anatomical study of Schlemm's canal and aqueous veins by means of neoprene casts II. Aqueous veins. Br J Ophthalmol 1952; 36:265–267.
19. Tripathi RC, Tripathi BJ. Functional anatomy of the anterior chamber angle. In: Duane TD, Jaeger EA, eds. Biomedical Foundations of Ophthalmology. Philadelphia: Lippincott; 1982.
20. Lütjen-Drecoll E. Functional morphology of the trabecular meshwork in primate eyes. Prog Ret Eye Res 1998; 18:91–119.
21. Mäepea O, Bill A. Pressures in the juxtacanalicular tissue and Schlemm's canal. Exp Eye Res 1992; 65:879–883.
22. Lee WR. The pathology of the outflow system in primary and secondary glaucoma. Eye 1995; 9:1–23.
23. Ethier CR. The inner wall of the canal of Schlemm. Exp Eye Res 2002; 74:161–172.
24. Grierson I, Lee WR. Light microscopic quantification of endothelial vacuoles in Schlemm's canal. Am J Ophthalmol 1977; 84:234–246.

25. Wiederholt M. Direct involvement of trabecular meshwork in the regulation of aqueous outflow. Curr Opin Ophthalmol 1998; 9:46–49.

26. Brubaker RF. Targeting outflow facility in glaucoma management. Surv Ophthalmol 2003; 48:S17–S20.

27. Bill A. The aqueous humor drainage mechanism in the cynomolgous monkey (*Macaca irus*) with evidence for unconventional routes. Invest Ophthalmol 965; 4:911–919.

Chapter 3

Histopathology and pathogenesis of glaucomatous optic neuropathy

John G Lawrenson

CHAPTER CONTENTS

3.1 INTRODUCTION

Since ophthalmoscopic observation of the optic nerve head (ONH) is fundamental to the diagnosis and management of glaucoma, it is important to be familiar not only with its gross anatomy but also with the histological appearance of those tissues that immediately underlie the disc. In this chapter particular emphasis will be placed on those aspects of the microscopic anatomy of the ONH that are most relevant to an understanding of the histopathology of glaucoma. It thus complements Chapter 9, which deals with the ophthalmoscopic features of the normal disc and the characteristic changes in glaucoma. In the final section, current theories for the pathogenesis of glaucomatous optic neuropathy will also be reviewed.

3.2 MICROSCOPIC APPEARANCE OF THE ONH

The ONH represents an area of considerable specialisation where axons from retinal ganglion cells leave the eye. The thickness of the nerve fibre layer increases from the periphery of the retina towards the disc, where it is elevated above the plane of the retina (giving rise to the alternative term for the disc 'optic papilla') (Fig. 3.1). Fibres from the nasal, superior and inferior retina follow a direct

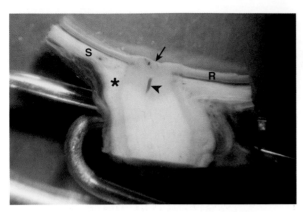

Fig. 3.1 Gross appearance of the optic nerve head sectioned longitudinally to show the optic cup (arrow), the central retinal vessels (arrow head) and the continuity between the sclera (S) and the dura mater (asterisk). R, retina. The paper clip gives an impression of the relative scale. (Courtesy of Gordon Ruskell.)

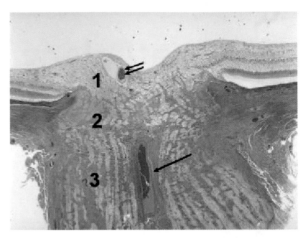

Fig. 3.2 Microscopic view of the ONH sectioned longitudinally. The pre-laminar (1), laminar (2) and post-laminar regions (3) are indicated. The central retinal artery is visible (arrow) and also branches of the central retinal vessels at the surface of the disc (double arrow).

course to the ONH. Fibres from the nasal side of the fovea (papillomacular bundle) also take a direct route. In contrast, axons from ganglion cells temporal to the fovea take arcuate paths to enter the ONH at its upper and lower margins. Axon bundles in the nerve head show a considerable degree of spatial order. Ganglion cells from the central retina generally have axons near the centre of the optic nerve; peripheral ganglion cells have axons near the periphery of the nerve.

At the ONH approximately one million ganglion cell axons leave the retina through the scleral canal. The outermost half of the sclera is reflected backwards to become continuous with the dura mater, and the innermost half is modified to form the lamina cribrosa (cribriform plate). The lamina cribrosa offers a conduit for retinal blood vessels and provides mechanical support for ganglion cell axons as they pass through the scleral canal. The lamina also serves as a convenient reference point for localisation purposes, and the terms 'pre-laminar', 'laminar' and 'post-laminar' are frequently used. Thus, when the nerve head is sectioned longitudinally it can be resolved into three distinct regions (Fig 3.2):

- Pre-laminar zone
- Laminar zone
- Post-laminar zone.

3.2.1 PRE-LAMINAR ZONE

At the interface with the vitreous, the ONH is covered by a canopy of astrocytes (the so-called internal limiting membrane of Elschnig) (Fig. 3.3). This membrane is thickened centrally and thins towards the periphery of the disc, where it is continuous with the inner limiting membrane of the retina. Within the pre-laminar region, fasciculation of axons is maintained by glial columns that extend forward from the lamina cribrosa. Further glial tissue is interposed between ONH axons and the choroid (border layer of Jacoby). This extends forward to form the intermediary tissue of Kuhnt, which separates ONH axons from the outer layers of the retina.[1,2]

3.2.2 LAMINAR ZONE

The lamina cribrosa consists of a meshwork formed by interlinked connective tissue plates (cribriform plates) principally composed of collagen types I, III, IV and elastin fibres. Central retinal vessels and bundles of axons pass through a series of round or oval apertures within the meshwork (Fig 3.4). The 300–400 pores that transmit axon bundles show a considerable variation in size, with the largest pores typically found in the superior and inferior

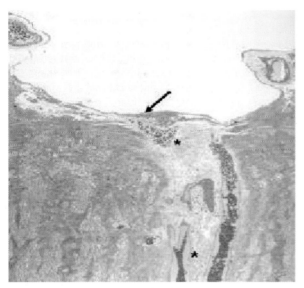

Fig. 3.3 Prelaminar ONH showing the canopy of astrocytes on the surface of the disc (arrowed). The central retinal vein and its branches are indicated (asterisks).

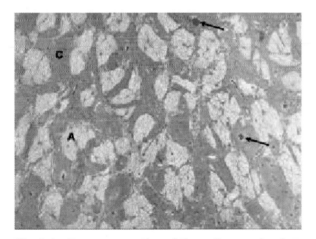

Fig. 3.4 Transverse section of the optic nerve head at the level of the lamina cribrosa. Pores between the collagen beams (C) are packed with unmyelinated axons (A) and astrocytes. The collagen beams contain numerous capillaries (arrowed).

quadrants. Within these regions the amount of connective tissue surrounding the pores is correspondingly reduced.[3] Each pore is lined by type 1A astrocytes that provide structural support and ensure that neural and connective tissue elements within the ONH are never in direct contact. In

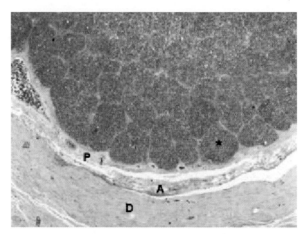

Fig. 3.5 Transverse section through the post-laminar ONH. The pia mater (P) is continuous with the septa that separate the optic nerve axons into fascicles (asterisk). The arachnoid mater (A) lies between the pia and the thick collagenous dura mater (D).

contrast, type 1B astrocytes are found throughout the ONH and are specialised for the physiological support of neurones by regulating the neural microenvironment.[4,5]

3.2.3 POST-LAMINAR ZONE

Axons within the post laminar optic nerve are myelinated, which principally accounts for the doubling of the optic nerve diameter from 1.5 mm at the pre-laminar and laminar levels to 3.0 mm in the post-laminar region. Oligodendrocytes, which are responsible for myelination of the nerve axons, are numerous. Unlike the Schwann cell of the peripheral nervous system, oligodendrocytes myelinate up to 40 axons, although only for a short length. Fasciculation of the myelinated nerve axons is maintained by connective tissue septa that are continuous with the lamina cribrosa. Within the post-laminar region meningeal sheaths invest the optic nerve: a thin pial layer, a middle arachnoid layer and a thick collagenous dural layer (Fig. 3.5).

3.3 BLOOD SUPPLY TO THE OPTIC NERVE HEAD

The regional variation of the ONH vasculature is complex (Fig. 3.6), and there is not yet complete

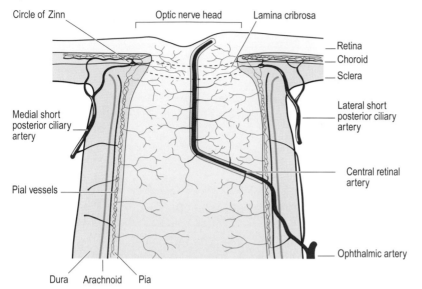

Fig. 3.6 Schematic representation of the arterial supply to the ONH. The pre-laminar zone is supplied by branches from the central retinal artery, and branches from the peripapillary choroid and short posterior ciliary arteries (SPCA). Centripetal branches from the SPCA or the circle of Zinn and Haller supply the laminar zone. Centripetal branches from the pia mater supply the post-laminar region.

agreement regarding the relative contribution from the various arterial sources.[6,7] The main source of arterial blood to the ONH is the posterior ciliary arteries, which derive from the ophthalmic artery. The number and site of entry of these arteries is variable, although typically two to three posterior ciliary arteries lie to the medial and lateral sides of the optic nerve. Prior to entering the sclera they divide into multiple smaller branches: 10–12 short posterior ciliary arteries (SPCAs) pierce the sclera close to the optic nerve, and one to two long posterior ciliary arteries penetrate further away. SPCAs contribute to an intrascleral arterial circle, the circle of Zinn and Haller, from which centripetal branches enter the laminar ONH (Fig. 3.7). The circle is typically supplied by either medial or lateral SPCAs and is frequently incomplete, indicating that the circle functions as an end-arterial system.[8]

The arterial supply to the ONH is segmental (see Fig. 3.6):

- Small branches from retinal arterioles and cilio-retinal arteries supply the superficial nerve fibre layer.
- Arterial branches from the peripapillary choroid and SPCAs supply the pre-laminar region.
- Centripetal branches from the SPCAs or the circle of Zinn supply the lamina cribrosa.
- Centripetal branches from the pia mater supply the post-laminar region.

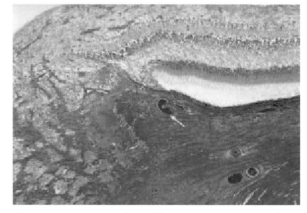

Fig. 3.7 Arterial circle of Zinn and Haller (arrowed). The circle is derived from branches of the short posterior ciliary arteries that traverse the sclera to supply the choroid.

Venous drainage occurs via the central retinal vein and there may also be some drainage into the peripapillary choroid.[7]

3.3.1 PHYSIOLOGY OF OPTIC NERVE HEAD BLOOD FLOW

Blood flow within the optic nerve head can be calculated from the following formula:[7]

Flow = Perfusion pressure/resistance to flow

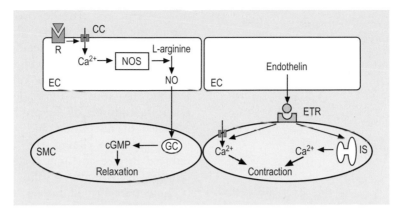

Fig. 3.8 Vascular endothelial cells (EC) release vasodilator molecules such as nitric oxide (NO) and vasoconstrictors such as endothelin-1 (ET-1) in response to the binding of agonists to membrane receptors (R) or mechanical forces on the vessel wall. NO release from EC activates guanyl cyclase (GC) in smooth muscle cells (SMC) leading to muscle relaxation. Endothelin binds to receptors (ETR), stimulating calcium intake through calcium channels (CC) and the release of calcium from internal stores (IS). Raised intracellular calcium is coupled to SMC constriction.

where perfusion pressure equals the mean arterial blood pressure (BP) in the ONH minus the intraocular pressure (IOP).

Thus the blood flow to the ONH depends on three parameters: (i) resistance to flow; (ii) BP; and (iii) IOP. The resistance to flow is the primary determinant of ONH perfusion, and is influenced principally by the calibre of the serving blood vessels and by blood viscosity. The principal resistance vessels within the vascular system are pre-capillary arterioles that regulate entry into the capillary bed; however there is evidence that pericytes may have a direct influence on capillary blood flow.[9] Within the ONH, tissue perfusion is maintained at a relatively constant level over a range of perfusion pressures. This process is termed 'autoregulation', and ensures that a constant supply of nutrients is available despite changes in mean arterial BP and IOP.[7] The exact mechanism responsible for autoregulation in the ONH is not fully understood. However, arteriolar smooth muscle and pericytes are responsive to alterations in the local concentrations of various metabolic products or changes in P_{O_2} and P_{CO_2} levels. Furthermore, a rise in intravascular pressure causes arteriolar vasoconstriction (myogenic response).[10] Recently, the importance of vascular endothelial-derived factors in the modulation of vascular tone and blood flow autoregulation has been

realised.[11,12] Vasoconstricting factors such as endothelin-1 (ET-1) or vasodilatory factors such as nitric oxide (NO) (Fig. 3.8) are released from vascular endothelial cells in response to the activation of membrane receptors or physical forces on the vessel wall. The balance between these opposing vasoactive modulators determines the state of contraction of vascular smooth muscle cells and pericytes and therefore ocular blood flow.[13]

3.4 THE OPTIC NERVE HEAD IN PRIMARY OPEN ANGLE GLAUCOMA

3.4.1 HISTOPATHOLOGY OF GLAUCOMATOUS OPTIC NEUROPATHY

Much of our knowledge of the histopathological changes in glaucoma comes from studies of animal models. Although these models largely address the IOP-mediated component of ONH damage, the observed morphological changes are very similar to those seen in human disease.[14] Open angle glaucoma is characterised by a slowly progressive loss of ganglion cells and their axons that is associated with excavation at the ONH, and thinning of the neuroretinal rim (Fig. 3.9). Many of the changes seen in primary open angle glaucoma (POAG) occur at the level of the lamina cribrosa. In human

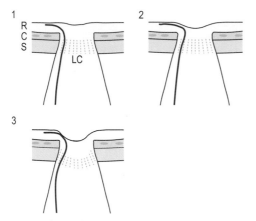

Fig. 3.9 Schematic representation showing the distortion of the lamina cribrosa in primary open angle glaucoma and progressive excavation of the ONH. Axon paths show greater deviation as the disease progresses. R, retina; C, choroid; S, sclera; LC, Lamina cribrosa.

eyes showing a moderate degree of field loss, compression of the connective tissue plates of the lamina cribrosa has been observed. With more severe field loss, this is associated with a rotation of the peripheral lamina cribrosa at its insertion into the sclera together with posterior bowing.[15] These changes potentially alter the paths taken by nerve axons as they course through the lamina (Fig. 3.9) and increase their susceptibility to damage. Electron microscopic observations have shown that axons at laminar level are swollen with intracellular organelles, and also show disorganisation of microtubules and neurofilaments. Studies of experimental glaucoma have suggested that these changes are caused by an obstruction of axon transport at laminar level.[16] Axon transport is an energy-dependent process that moves neuronal components from the cell body to sites of utilisation along the axon and its terminals (anterograde transport). Moreover, neurotrophic substances are taken up at presynaptic terminals and transported back to the cell body (retrograde transport). Ultimately impaired axon transport leads to retinal ganglion cell dysfunction and death. Neuronal cell death in glaucoma appears to be specific to retinal ganglion cells and the remainder of the inner retina and outer retina remains largely unaffected.[17] However, non-neuronal cells within the retina and the ONH also show evidence of disruption and altered func-

tion. Astrocytes are the predominant glial cell within the ONH and are vital for ganglion cell health. Since they are metabolically very active, astrocytes are particularly vulnerable to physiological perturbations, and are often the first cell to respond to injury.[4] In glaucomatous eyes, the astrocyte columns of the pre-laminar ONH show evidence of disruption and atrophy. At laminar level, astrocytes lining the cribrosal pores are reduced in size and migrate into the nerve fibre bundles. Throughout the ONH, astrocytes become transformed into a 'reactive' phenotype that release potential neurotoxins and also show an altered synthetic profile. It is likely therefore that astrocyte dysfunction plays an important role in the initiation of axon damage, and may also contribute to the extracellular matrix changes seen within the ONH in glaucoma.[4,18]

3.4.2 PATHOGENESIS OF GLAUCOMATOUS OPTIC NEUROPATHY: MECHANICAL VERSUS VASOGENIC THEORIES

The selective nature of the visual field loss and other aspects of visual function in glaucoma, would suggest that not all ganglion cells are compromised simultaneously. Ganglion cell death shows a characteristic spatial and temporal pattern that depends on the magnitude of the insult. In recent years the view has been popularised that ganglion cells with a large cell soma and axon (magno (M) cells) are selectively damaged in early POAG.[14] However, this interpretation has been questioned by several authors[19] who argue that the smaller parvo (P) cells also sustain early damage. The precise mechanism for the initiation of ganglion cell dysfunction in POAG remains elusive, despite extensive research. A number of explanatory theories have been suggested that can be grouped into two broad categories: mechanical (or IOP-mediated) and vasogenic,[20] although it is becoming increasingly apparent that the disease possesses a complex and multifactorial aetiology (Fig. 3.10).

Mechanical

The mechanical theory suggests that axon damage within the ONH is induced by pressure-induced deformation of the lamina cribrosa leading to

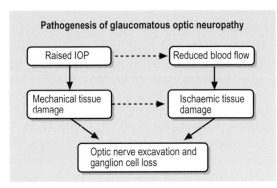

Fig. 3.10 Diagram showing the interplay of mechanical and vasogenic mechanisms in the pathogenesis of primary open angle glaucoma.

blockage of axon transport.[14] Support for this mechanism comes from a variety of sources:

- When IOP is experimentally raised to a sufficiently high level and for a sufficient amount of time, an optic neuropathy develops that is histopathologically indistinguishable from human POAG.[3]
- In patients with normal tension glaucoma (NTG) and asymmetrical IOPs the eye with the higher IOP tends to show the greatest field loss.[21]
- Optic disc cupping has been shown to reduce following a reduction in IOP.[22]
- Randomised controlled trials in glaucoma have shown a beneficial effect of lowering IOP on visual function.[23]

The lamina cribrosa represents a weak point within the tough outer coat of the globe, and is thus vulnerable to the effects of raised IOP. Although IOP-mediated forces should be distributed evenly across the lamina, it appears that variation in the proportion of supporting connective tissue may lead to selective weakening and distortion at the upper and lower poles.[14] Increased distortion within these regions would lead to a greater deviation of axon paths as they course through the lamina, increasing the risk of mechanical damage.[5] The preferential pattern of axon damage seen at the ONH in POAG is consistent with this notion.[14] However, glaucomatous excavation at the ONH is also seen in a proportion of patients with IOPs within the normal range. It has

been speculated that in these cases the lamina cribrosa may possess connective tissue abnormalities that account for its susceptibility to injury.

Vasogenic

According to the vasogenic theory, raised IOP may also disturb the quality of the blood supply to the ONH, leading to hypoxia and reduced nutrition to optic nerve axons,[18] which ultimately leads to ganglion cell death. Alterations in the quality of the blood supply to the optic nerve head can also be induced by factors that are independent of IOP, e.g. reduced arterial blood pressure, increased blood viscosity, local vasospasm or altered autoregulation.[7] Although in a clinical setting it is not possible to measure ocular blood flow (OBF) directly, using indirect methods abnormalities in OBF have been described in patients with POAG, especially those with NTG (reviewed by Flammer et al[24]). There is sufficient evidence to assume that this reduction in OBF is a pathogenic event, rather than a secondary effect of the disease itself. Although increased IOP alone is sufficient to induce glaucomatous damage, either by mechanical or vasogenic mechanisms, nerve damage can occur in patients who have never previously demonstrated elevated IOP, and some patients show glaucomatous progression despite normalisation of IOP. In such patients, it is likely that vascular factors play a major role. However, the beneficial effects of IOP reduction in NTG suggest that there is an interplay between risk factors.[25] The mainstay of treatment for POAG remains ocular hypotensive drugs. Although these agents can improve ocular perfusion dynamics indirectly, future therapy may more specifically address vascular dysfunction to improve blood flow within the ONH.

3.4.3 MECHANISMS OF GANGLION CELL DEATH

Regardless of the mechanism of injury, the final common pathway in POAG is retinal ganglion cell death with resulting irreversible visual field loss.[26] Evidence from animal models and human POAG indicates that ganglion cells die by a process of apoptosis.[27] Apoptosis is a form of programmed cell death, where a genetically coded 'suicide' programme is activated when cells are no longer needed, or in response to various stress stimuli.[28] A wide variety of such stimuli can trigger apoptosis, but in the context of glaucoma the most important are:

Ischaemia: Neurones are dependent on oxidative metabolism for their survival. Following an ischaemic insult a variety of events can lead to neuronal death including ATP depletion and free radical damage.[17]

Excitotoxicity: The toxicity of glutamate to retinal ganglion cells is well documented, and high levels of glutamate have been found in the vitreous humour of patients with glaucoma.[29] Glutamate exerts its toxic effects through activation of the *N*-methyl-D-aspartate (NMDA) membrane receptor. Stimulation of the receptor by glutamate induces an influx of extracellular calcium that in turn activates intracellular pathways leading to apoptosis.

Withdrawal of trophic support: Neurones are dependent for their survival on the retrograde transport of soluble factors, termed neurotrophins, from the nerve terminal to the cell soma. The neurotrophin that has attracted the most attention is brain-derived neurotrophic factor (BDNF).[30] Since the interruption of axon transport at the lamina cribrosa is a hallmark of glaucomatous optic neuropathy, it is conceivable that retrograde transport of neurotrophins such as brain-derived growth factor (BDGF) could be impeded which may contribute to ganglion cell death.[26]

There is currently a great deal of interest in finding novel therapies for the treatment of POAG. An understanding of the cellular and molecular events associated with ganglion cell death in glaucoma will ultimately lead to the development of neuroprotective therapies that can be used in combination with a traditional IOP-lowering approach.

References

1. Anderson DR, Hoyt WF. Ultrastructure of the intraorbital portion of the human and monkey optic nerve. Arch Ophthalmol 1969; 82:506–530.
2. Anderson DR, Hoyt WF, Hogan MJ. The fine structure of the astroglia in the human optic nerve and optic nerve head. Trans Ophthalmol Soc 1967; 65:275–305.
3. Quigley HA, Addicks EM. Regional differences in the structure of the lamina cribrosa and their relation to glaucomatous optic nerve damage. Arch Ophthalmol 1981; 99:137–143.
4. Morgan JE. Optic nerve head structure in glaucoma: astrocytes as mediators of axon damage. Eye 2000; 14:437–444.
5. Morgan JE. Circulation and axon transport on the optic nerve. Eye 2004; 18:1089–1095.
6. Lieberman MF, Shahi A, Green WR. Histologic studies of the vasculature of the anterior optic nerve. Am J Ophthalmol 1976; 82:405–423.
7. Hayreh SS. Blood flow in the optic nerve head and factors that may influence it. Prog Ret Eye Res 2001; 20:595–624.
8. Ruskell GL. Blood flow in the Zinn-Haller circle. Br J Ophthalmol 1998; 82:1351–1353.
9. Allt G, Lawrenson JG. Pericytes: Cell Biology and Pathology. Cells Tiss Org 2001; 169:1–11.
10. Levick JR. An introduction to cardiovascular physiology, 3rd edn. London: Arnold; 2000.
11. Orgül S, Gugleta K, Flammer J. Physiology of perfusion as it relates to the optic nerve head. Surv Ophthalmol 1999; 43:S17–S26.
12. Grieshaber MC, Flammer J. Blood flow in glaucoma. Curr Opin Ophthalmol 2005; 16:79–83.
13. Haefliger IO, Flammer J, Bény JL, et al. Endothelial-dependent vasoactive modulation in the ophthalmic circulation. Prog Ret Eye Res 2001; 20:209–225.
14. Quigley HA. Neuronal death in glaucoma. Prog Ret Eye Res 2001; 18:39–57.
15. Quigley HA, Hohman RM, Addicks EM, et al. Morphological changes in the lamina cribrosa correlated with neural loss in open angle glaucoma. Am J Ophthalmol 1983; 95:673–691.
16. Minckler DS, Bunt AH, Johanson GW. Orthograde and retrograde axoplasmic transport during acute ocular hypertension in the monkey. Invest Ophthalmol Vis Sci 1977; 16:426–441.
17. Osborne NN, Ugarte M, Chao M, et al. Neuroprotection in relation to retinal ischaemia and relevance to glaucoma. Surv Ophthalmol 1999; 43:S102–S128.

18. Osborne NN, Melena J, Chidlow G, et al. A hypothesis to explain ganglion cell death caused by vascular insults at the optic nerve head: possible implications for the treatment of glaucoma. Br J Ophthalmol 2001; 85:1252–1259.

19. Morgan JE. Selective cell death in glaucoma: does it really occur? Br J Ophthalmol 1994; 78:875–880.

20. Fechtner RD, Weiner RN. Mechanisms of optic nerve damage in primary open angle glaucoma. Surv Ophthalmol 1994; 39:23–42.

21. Cartwright MJ, Anderson DR. Correlation of asymmetrical damage with asymmetrical intraocular pressure in normal tension glaucoma. Arch Ophthalmol 1998; 106:898–900.

22. Lusky M, Morsman D, Weinreb RN. Effect of intraocular pressure reduction on optic nerve head topography. Curr Opin Ophthalmol 1993; 4:40–45.

23. Maier PG, Funk J, Schwarzer G, et al. Treatment of ocular hypertension and open angle glaucoma: meta-analysis of randomised controlled trials. BMJ 2005; 331:134–136.

24. Flammer J, Orgül S, Costa VP, et al. The impact of ocular blood flow in glaucoma. Prog Ret Eye Res 2002, 21:359–393,

25. Collaborative Normal-Tension Glaucoma Study Group. The effectiveness of intraocular pressure reduction in the treatment of normal tension glaucoma. Am J Ophthalmol 1998; 126:498–505.

26. McKinnon SJ. Glaucoma, apoptosis and neuroprotection. Curr Opin Ophthalmol 1997; 8:28–37.

27. Kerrigan LA, Zack DJ, Quigley HA, et al. TUNEL-positive ganglion cells in human primary open angle glaucoma. Arch Ophthalmol 1997; 115:1031–1035.

28. Nickells RW. Apoptosis of retinal ganglion cells in glaucoma: an update of molecular pathways involved in cell death. Surv Ophthalmol 1999; 43:S151–S161.

29. Dreyer EB, Zurakowski D, Schumer RA, et al. Elevated glutamate levels in the vitreous body of humans and monkeys with glaucoma. Arch Ophthalmol 1996; 114:299 305.

30. Naskar R, Dreyer EB New horizons in neuroprotection. Surv Ophthalmol 2001; 45:S250–S255.

Chapter 4

Evaluation of the anterior chamber angle

C Lisa Prokopich and John G Flanagan

CHAPTER CONTENTS

4.1 INTRODUCTION

Evaluation of the anterior chamber angle is an essential component in the clinical assessment of the glaucoma patient or suspect. This chapter will consist of an outline of the relevant clinical techniques, concentrating mainly on gonioscopy, along with a guide to interpretation of the findings. The congenital and developmental glaucomas will not be considered as they would not normally be included within a co-management arrangement or be managed by a primary eye care clinician.

Gonioscopy refers to the technique used to view and define the structures and abnormalities of the anterior chamber or iridocorneal angle.[1-6] Improvements to gonioscopic lenses and techniques have made the procedure accessible and more feasible in the primary eye care examination. Detection of narrow angles by the van Herick method (Table 4.1) is one of the indications for evaluating a patient's angles to determine the risk for spontaneous and pharmacologically induced angle closure.[7] All patients determined to be at risk for primary or secondary open or closed angle glaucoma should have gonioscopy performed to identify further risk factors, and to differentiate the disease aetiology and decide the most appropriate therapeutic approach (Table 4.2). Gonioscopy should also be performed periodically on every chronic glaucoma patient to monitor detectable changes to the drainage structures.

Gonioscopy is contraindicated following acute trauma especially in the presence of hyphaema or

Table 4.1   **van Herick slit lamp angle grading system**

Grade	Comparison of corneal section width to shadow formed in angle	Likelihood of primary (pupillary block) angle closure (with or without mydriatic agents)
4	1:1 or 1:>1	Not likely
3	1:1/4 to 1:1/2*	Not likely
2	1:1/4	Angle is considered capable of angle closure
1	1:<1/4	Angle closure likely
Slit-like	Very little shadow seen	Angle closure imminent
Closed[†]	No shadow seen	Angle is closed

* Angles wider than 1:1/2 but less than 1:1 may be designated Grade 3+, or Grade 4−.

[†] Note that eyes with arcus should not necessarily be interpreted as closed if no shadow is seen.

Table 4.2   **Indications for gonioscopy in glaucoma[3,4,6]**

Type	Indications	Specific indications Primary glaucomas
Open angle	All glaucoma patients	Gonioscopy is essential to determine the mechanism of glaucoma, e.g. primary vs. type of secondary *Primary open angle glaucoma is a diagnosis of exclusion*
	All glaucoma suspect patients	Elevated intraocular pressure (IOP) (>21 mmHg) IOP asymmetry of ≥3 mmHg Suspicious optic nerve head appearance and/or asymmetry of the optic disc cups Multifactorial risk factors: e.g. suspicious visual field defects, positive family history, vasospastic disease and anaemias, nutritional abnormalities, myopia, diabetes, race, age
Closed angle	Narrow angle and shallow anterior chamber	van Herick grade 2 angle assessment or narrower Other anatomical features often associated with the narrow angle, e.g. hyperopia, short axial length, shallow anterior chamber, small corneal diameter, steep corneal curvature, thicker crystalline lens, anterior lens position
	Suspicion of plateau iris configuration	Narrow angle by van Herick but deep anterior chamber
	Mild forms of angle closure: intermittent and sub-acute	Brief relative pupillary block episodes that resolve spontaneously (often lead to an acute attack) Uniocular dull ache, mild blurry vision, rarely haloes, recurrences at same time of day or following near work Symptoms often reported to be relieved by sleep
	Chronic and creeping angle closure	Uncommon in Caucasians, common in Asians, tends to occur in Afro-Caribbeans who develop angle closure Asymptomatic repeated attacks cause portions of the angle to be permanently closed by peripheral anterior synechiae Often lead to an acute attack

Table 4.2   Continued

Type	Indications	Specific indications Primary glaucomas
	Acute angle closure	Precipitating events include illness, emotional stress, trauma, intense concentration, pupillary dilation (pharmacological or physiological) Blurred vision, haloes, intense pain, ciliary injection, lid oedema, tearing, anxiety, fatigue, nausea, mid-dilated/vertically oval pupil

Type	Indications	Specific indications Secondary glaucomas
Open angle		Pigment dispersion (PDS): endothelial pigment deposition (often Krukenberg spindle), iris transillumination defects, heavy pigment deposition in angle Pseudoexfoliation syndrome (PEX): flaky debris noted on iris frill and in bulls eye pattern (visible on lens once pupil is dilated), pigment clumping in angle Iridocorneal endothelial syndromes (ICE syndromes): down growth of endothelial cells over trabeculum, polycoria or irregular pupil (usually unilateral) with or without monocular diplopia Corticosteroid induced from chronic use of topical steroid drops Recurrent or chronic inflammation (anterior uveitis): cells in anterior chamber with or without flare, including Fuchs iridocyclitis, glaucomatocyclitic crisis (Posner–Schlossmann syndrome), phakolytic and systemic disease associated uveitis Non-acute history of ocular trauma: concern of angle recession, cyclodialysis, suspicion of intraocular foreign body Blood-induced post surgery or trauma, e.g. ghost cell, haemolytic, hemosiderotic glaucoma Elevated episcleral venous pressure: venous obstruction (e.g. thyroid ophthalmopathy), or arteriovenous anomaly (e.g. carotid cavernous sinus fistula) Drug-induced: some drugs have been shown to increase IOP (uncommon)
Closed angle	Anterior mechanism: angle is *pulled* closed	Risk of rubeosis iridis and neovascular glaucoma (NVG secondary to ischaemic retinal disease), iridocorneal endothelial syndromes (ICE), posterior polymorphous dystrophy Risk of peripheral anterior synechiae following trauma and/or inflammation (anterior uveitis)
	Posterior mechanism: angle is *pushed* closed	Lens related: thickened intumescent lens, forward subluxation Iris and ciliary body cysts or tumours Pseudophakic pupillary block Malignant glaucoma Retina–choroid related: choroidal effusion (e.g. following panretinal photocoagulation, scleral buckling, intravitreal gas injection or silicone, pars plana vitrectomy, and has been reported in AIDS)
	Uncommon causes	Certain drugs (e.g. psychotropics, antidepressants, antihistamines, antiparkinsonian agents, autonomic agents) that cause pupillary dilation may precipitate chronic angle closure in susceptible individuals Intraocular tumours: uveal melanomas, metastatic tumours, retinoblastoma, phakomatoses Retinal related: e.g. central retinal vein occlusion (rare)

microhyphaema. Seidel's test is indicated when an intraocular foreign body is suspected and B-scan ultrasonography or X-ray should also be considered to rule out foreign body penetration. Similarly, gonioscopy is not recommended immediately post-cataract surgery or following other penetrating intraocular surgeries.

4.2 METHODS OF EXAMINATION

Light rays from the anterior drainage structures form an angle greater than the critical angle that would permit direct imaging of structural detail. Therefore the majority of light returning from the angle is totally internally reflected at the tear–air interface into the anterior chamber (Fig. 4.1) and the angle structures cannot be viewed directly with the biomicroscope alone. Only when the corneal power is neutralised with a plus contact lens (direct) or contact mirror system (indirect) can the structures be visualised. The direct technique uses a high plus (+50D Koeppe) lens[5] that must be used

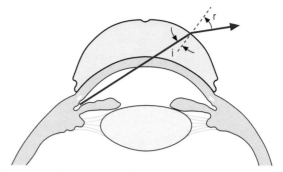

Fig. 4.2 Direct (Koeppe) gonioscope on cornea. Light from the angle is refracted laterally and must be viewed with a hand-held illuminated magnifier.

in conjunction with a hand-held slit lamp or other magnifying instrument despite the 1.5× magnification it provides, as the patient must be in the reclined position. Advantages include a panoramic undistorted view of 360° of the angle and the ability to compare the angles of both eyes simultaneously when a lens is inserted in each eye.[8] The Koeppe lens is rarely used in the modern primary care practice and is generally limited to the examination of infants or children under general anaesthesia or prior to anterior chamber angle surgery (Fig. 4.2).

Indirect gonioscopic lenses provide the method of choice in the routine assessment of the glaucoma suspect or patient.[9] There are many types of indirect lens[10] (see Table 4.3) with mirrors mounted within the lens carrier angled between 59° and 64°. The mirror reflects light from the anterior chamber angle through the front of the lens (Fig. 4.3). This permits a stereoscopic view of the structures within the angle assisted by the magnification and illumination options of the slit lamp biomicroscope. The principle of the gonioscopy contact lens is that the corneal surface is approximately neutralised by the rear surface of the contact lens and the tears formed between this surface and the cornea. A clear coupling fluid is usually used to facilitate contact (see Table 4.4). The image of the angle is in the opposite quadrant to the position of the mirror and forms a reversed image.

The indirect methods have a number of advantages, not the least of which is the ease of use while the patient is seated at the slit lamp and therefore facilitation of the application of laser in procedures

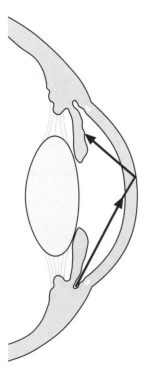

Fig. 4.1 Light from the anterior chamber angle exceeds the critical angle and is totally internally reflected.

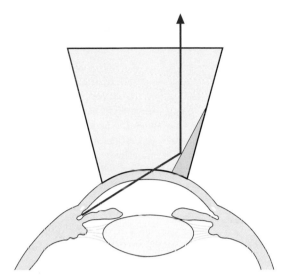

Fig. 4.3 Indirect gonioscope placed on cornea. Light from the opposite angle is reflected from the internal mirror to the front of the lens where the reversed image is viewed with a slit lamp.

such as trabeculoplasty. Focal line and convex iris techniques (see Additional examination techniques) can be performed with these lenses to facilitate diagnostic examination, and compression can be used as a therapeutic technique in angle closure. Disadvantages of the indirect techniques will be discussed in the following section on the lens types.

4.3 TYPES OF INDIRECT GONIOSCOPES[10] (Fig. 4.4)

Two basic types of gonioscope are available which will be designated here as scleral-type and corneal type lenses because of the contact area of the lenses on the eye. Scleral-type lenses have a broad area of contact and a steep concave surface. A viscous solution must be used to fill the gap between the lens and the cornea in order to obtain an image through the lens. Scleral lenses are available in a range of sizes (including lenses designed for children) with a typical diameter of 15 mm or 18 mm. The most commonly used lens is the Goldmann-type 3-mirror or 'Universal' lens. This lens affords the clinician the further advantage of having two other mirrors (more steeply angled than the gonioscopy or 'thumb-nail' shaped mirror) as well as a central lens to allow stereoscopic evaluation of all areas of the vitreous and retina. Other available lenses include 1, 2 and 4-mirror types.[5,9]

Scleral-type lenses are most commonly used for gonioscopy. Advantages include excellent optics and lens and lid stabilisation even with a blepharospastic patient. The procedure also causes very little if any corneal disruption when a non-preserved coupling solution (such as Celluvisc™) is used. Alternatively, a commercially available gonioscopic solution may be considered for its increased viscosity; however, these solutions are preserved with either benzalkonium chloride or thimerosal (thiomersal) and must be rinsed from the eye to prevent corneal disruption and staining. Because of the wide area of contact, scleral-type lenses cannot be used for indentation (compression) gonioscopy. When the lens is centred, the mirror is located approximately 7 mm from the apex of the cornea so the examiner's technique may need to be altered to view over a convex iris. The focal line or slit technique used to locate Schwalbe's line in a narrow or difficult-to-assess angle can be performed most easily with scleral-type lenses (see Additional examination techniques).

All corneal-type lenses (Zeiss, Posner, Sussman) have four mirrors, generally angled at 64°. The Zeiss lens has a removable handle used to stabilise the lens. The Posner is a lighter version with a permanently attached handle that is angled away from the lens to facilitate manipulation. The Sussman is a hand-held version of the other two. Because the area of contact of corneal lenses is much smaller (9 mm) and the surface is similar in curvature to the cornea, the clinician is more likely to indent the cornea causing folds in Descemet's membrane with very little pressure. This may also cause the clinician to dangerously misinterpret the angle to be artificially wider as the peripheral iris and ciliary body will bow backward with pressure. An advantage of the corneal lens is the deliberate use of the indentation technique to differentiate an appositional- versus a synechial-type angle closure. In addition, the view over a convex iris is facilitated because the mirror is placed approximately 3 mm from the apex of the cornea.

Corneal lenses are easier and faster to use for the experienced gonioscopist. The four mirrors allow a

Table 4.3 Common gonioscopic lenses[9]

Lens	Type of indirect lens	Gonioscopic solution	Number of gonioscopic mirrors	Comments
Goldmann 3-mirror	Scleral	Yes	1	59° mirror for gonioscopy and far peripheral examination, along with 2 additional mirrors with steeper angles to examine the peripheral (66–67°) and mid-peripheral (73°) retina. Also a central lens for posterior pole examination Available in a variety of sizes down to paediatric 10 mm aperture. Ora serrata attachment available
Goldmann 4-mirror	Scleral	Yes	1	As with the 3-mirror with an additional mirror for retinal examination
1- and 2-mirror lenses	Scleral	Yes	1–2	Smaller lenses that are easier to insert in patients with small lid aperture
Thorpe type	Scleral	Yes	4	No rotation required to view different quadrants, no retinal mirrors
Zeiss	Corneal	No*	4	No rotation required to view different quadrants, handle is removable, compression gonioscopy possible
Posner	Corneal	No*	4	No rotation required to view different quadrants, attached handle is angled to facilitate stabilisation, compression gonioscopy possible
Sussman	Corneal	No*	4	No rotation required to view different quadrants, no handle so is held much like an indirect retinal lens, compression gonioscopy possible

* A viscous solution is not required but examination is facilitated by good optical contact; a viscous solution such as Celluvisc is therefore recommended.

Table 4.4[11] Gonioscopic coupling solutions

Solution	Supplier	Polymer	Preservative
Gonioscopic™	Alcon	Hydroxyethylcellulose	Thimerosal 0.004% edetate disodium 0.1%
Goniosol™	Iolab	Hydroxypropylmethylcellulose 2.5%	Benzalkonium chloride 0.01% edetate disodium
Gonak™	Akorn	Hydroxypropylmethylcellulose 2.5%	Benzalkonium chloride 0.01%
Celluvisc™ (recommended)	Allergan	Carboxymethylcellulose 1% unit dose containers	Preservative free

Approximately a third to half of the reservoir should be filled with solution and be free of bubbles which will interfere with the mirror view. Too much solution will cause some of it to run down the patient's cheek during examination, and too little will cause bubbles in the solution which will block the view of the angle. Gonioscopic, Gonak, and Goniosol are commercially available solutions which provide a clear medium and enable good contact suction with scleral-type lenses. These solutions must be irrigated from the eye after the lens has been removed to minimise irritation and corneal stippling from the large polymer and preservative. Rotation of the lens is most easily accomplished with these solutions. A viable alternative is a viscous unpreserved artifical tear solution such as Celluvisc (carboxymethylcellulose) as it can be used from one single dose vial and need not be rinsed from the eye. Rotation of the lens is marginally more difficult.

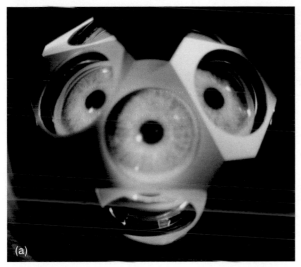

Fig. 4.4a 3-mirror (Goldmann or Universal) scleral-type lens. Thumbnail gonioscopic mirror positioned inferiorly.

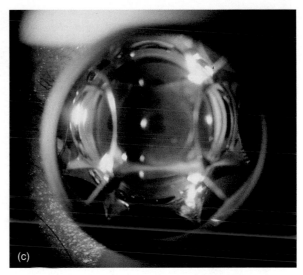

Fig. 4.4c 4-mirror (Sussman) corneal-type lens.

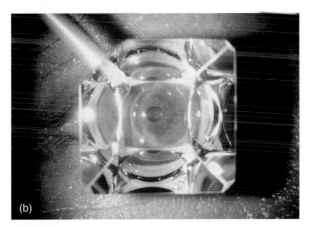

Fig. 4.4b 4-mirror (Posner) corneal-type lens (also very similar to the Zeiss lens).

view of all quadrants by manipulation of the slit lamp only. Examination may be somewhat discontinuous, however, and this can be important when evaluating the angle for suspected abnormalities such as angle recession or neovascularisation. The view of the angle structures is also not as optically distinct or stable as with the scleral lenses so that observation of subtleties and use of the focal line technique are more difficult. Along with folds in Descemet's membrane occurring with excessive pressure, corneal abrasions may occasionally occur

especially in patients with a compromised epithelium. Corneal lenses are very difficult to use in blepharospastic or uncooperative patients.

4.4 TECHNIQUES FOR INDIRECT GONIOSCOPY

Insertion and manipulation of the two main types of indirect lenses, the scleral- and corneal-type lenses, varies according to the lens characteristics (Table 4.5). In both cases, position the patient at the biomicroscope with the illumination coaxial with the viewing system and magnification low (10×). Ensure appropriate alignment with the lateral canthal marker so that the vertical range of the slit lamp is centred and therefore the mirrors may be viewed in all positions without altering the chin rest (Fig. 4.5). Describe the procedure and necessity for angle observation.

4.5 GONIOSCOPIC ANATOMY AND INTERPRETATION (Fig. 4.6)

The examiner must understand the relation between the structures of the iridocorneal angle so that variations and abnormalities can be identified. It is useful to approach the angle evaluation from

Table 4.5   Indirect gonioscopic technique

Scleral-type lenses	Corneal-type lenses
Preparation	
Position patient at biomicroscope with illumination coaxial with viewing system and magnification low (10×). Ensure appropriate alignment with lateral canthal marker and therefore vertical range of slit lamp	Position patient at biomicroscope with illumination coaxial with viewing system and magnification low (10×). Ensure appropriate alignment with lateral canthal marker and therefore vertical range of slit lamp
Clean/disinfect lens surface*	Clean/disinfect lens surface*
Lubricate lens with unpreserved (Celluvisc) solution or commercially available gonioscopic solution (Table 4.4) Support elbow on table/tissue boxes or, once lens is on, with little finger hooked on headrest	Consider lubricating lens with a drop of saline, anaesthetic, or Celluvisc. Forearm must be fully supported
Anaesthetise both the testing eye as well as the non-testing eye to minimise blink reflex	Anaesthetise both the testing eye as well as the non-testing eye to minimise blink reflex
Lens insertion	
Have patient look up and stabilise the upper lid against the brow bone. Pull the lower lid down and introduce the rim of the lens onto the inferior bulbar conjunctiva above the lower lid margin	Have patient look straight ahead and place the lens directly onto the apical surface so that the edges do not indent the cornea
Use lens edge to pull down lower lid further then quickly and gently rotate the lens onto the eye	Use backs of fingers to stabilise on cheek
Ask patient to *slowly* look straight ahead	Have lens such that the mirrors are placed in the 12, 6, 3 and 9 o'clock positions ('square'). Zeiss and Posner lens handles can be held in either superior or inferior temporal orientations
It is helpful (but not necessary) to manipulate the lens through a couple of rotations while maintaining sufficient pressure. The suction seal will noticeably 'loosen'	Maintain minimal contact to eliminate air beneath the surface. Watch for folds in Descemet's membrane indicating excessive pressure
Ensure no bubbles have entered behind the lens (if peripheral bubbles have entered, apply pressure to the opposite side of the lens to try to work them out. If large central bubbles have entered such that an image cannot be obtained, remove the lens and reinsert)	
Lens manipulation	
Hold lens between thumb and second finger (first finger should be free)	Manipulation is not usually necessary due to the four mirror configuration, i.e. only the slit lamp beam need be moved between the four mirrors
Rotate lens by placing first finger on the front of lens and using as a pivot while adjusting the second finger and thumb (this method allows freedom of the other hand to manipulate the slit lamp therefore facilitating an efficient exam where the examiner need not leave the eyepieces or use two hands to turn the lens)	Minimal lens tilting can be used to visualise the most posterior structure
	Indentation (or compression) gonioscopy can be used to differentiate an appositional vs. synechial angle closure

Table 4.5   Continued

Scleral-type lenses	Corneal-type lenses
Viewing	
Use vertical parallelopiped beam ~2–3 mm wide	As per Goldmann
The quadrant *opposite* the mirror is being viewed	Viewing over a convex iris is more difficult as the edge of the lens comes in contact with the cornea if the patient is asked to look toward the mirror. Some tilting can be used, however, to facilitate the view of a narrow angle
Start with inferior angle (place mirror superiorly) as it is the widest and usually has more pigmentation to highlight structures	
Maintain the parallelopiped in the mirror by manipulating the joystick of the slit lamp to follow the rotating mirror	
Examine all quadrants in a systematic manner	
Angles on the nasal and temporal sides may be more easily viewed when the slit beam is on the viewing axis (i.e. horizontal)	
Use convex iris technique for narrow angle/bowed iris	
Lens removal	
Release suction of the lens by having the patient look toward their nose and blink (strongest lid force nasally) while simultaneously applying pressure through the temporal inferior lid margin along the lens edge to introduce air beneath the lens. When the suction is broken the lens may make a popping sound and should fall forward. Repeat with more pressure temporally if first attempt fails. Do not use pulling force to remove the lens	Simply release from eye
	Wash lens with soap and water and dry before storing
Wash lens with soap and water and dry before storing	
Irrigation	
Rinse the superior and inferior cul-de-sacs with irrigating solution (or saline) to prevent blurred vision or discomfort if and only if a preserved coupling solution was used	Not required
Corneal assessment	
Check cornea for staining/disruption	Check cornea for staining/disruption

* A thorough soap and water wash on lens removal followed by a 10-minute soak in either a 1:10 dilution of hypochlorite (bleach) or fresh hydrogen peroxide with sterile saline rinse is the most appropriate disinfection of the contact surfaces of the lens. Alcohol has been used routinely in the past but, when used appropriately with surface rubbing, can cause damage to the lens surface with time.

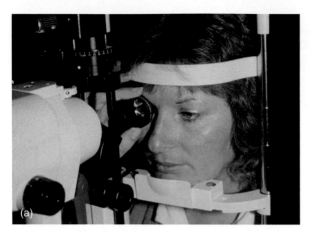

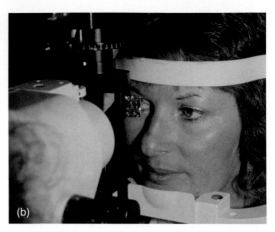

Fig. 4.5a   Scleral-type (Goldmann) lens must be rotated 360° to view all quadrants.

Fig. 4.5b   With corneal-type lens (Posner or Zeiss) only the slit lamp joystick needs be altered to view all quadrants.

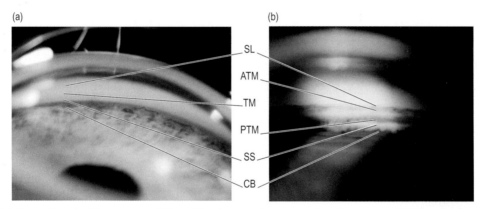

Fig. 4.6   (a) Normal angle (Caucasian), diffuse illumination, low magnification. A very lightly pigmented angle. The faintly gray trabecular meshwork (TM) band is just distinguishable above the dark ciliary body (CB) with scleral spur (SS) in between. A normal vessel is seen, and this is common in patients with lighter uveae. (b) Normal angle (Asian-Oriental), parallelopiped, high magnification. A more heavily pigmented angle. Pigment is evident on Schwalbe's line (SL), below which are seen the anterior (unpigmented) trabecular meshwork (ATM) then the posterior (pigmented) trabecular meshwork (PTM). A bright scleral spur is seen between the PTM and the blackish colour of the ciliary body. Small iris (or ciliary) processes are seen inserting onto the ciliary body.

an *anterior-to-posterior* direction to avoid misinterpretation especially when narrowness and angle variations and abnormalities complicate the textbook appearance. The anatomical structures seen in an open angle (from anterior to posterior) begin at the termination of the cornea at Schwalbe's line, followed by the trabecular meshwork and then scleral spur. The ciliary body, often the most conspicuous structure, is the most posteriorly viewed structure if the angle is widely open.[1-6,8-11]

4.5.1 SCHWALBE'S LINE

Schwalbe's line is a condensation of connective tissue that represents the termination of

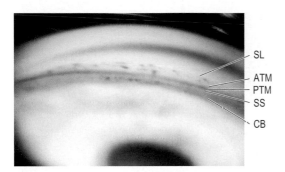

Fig. 4.7 Discontinuous pigmentation deposited in the angle is commonly seen in pseudoexfoliation syndrome. Pigmentation on Schwalbe's line is termed Sampaolesi's line. See Fig. 4.6 legend for abbreviations.

Descemet's membrane or end of the cornea. The appearance of Schwalbe's line is variable but it is a crucial landmark in interpreting the angle configuration. Schwalbe's line is often indistinguishable by direct observation but may be identified using the focal line technique. It may appear as a fine bright white line in some regions of the angle, as a shelf protruding into the anterior chamber, or it may have pigment deposited along it. Pigment deposited in a wavy discontinuous pattern anterior to SL is referred to as **Sampaolesi's line** and has been described in pseudoexfoliation syndrome (see Fig. 4.7). **Posterior embryotoxon** is a prominent SL that extends into the anterior chamber and is often visible directly with the slit lamp as a white line at the temporal limbus.

4.5.2 TRABECULAR MESHWORK

The anterior translucent portion of the trabecular meshwork (ATM) is considered the non filtering portion of the meshwork. The more posterior and usually more pigmented portion (PTM) overlies the **canal of Schlemm** and is more active in the drainage of aqueous. Aqueous fluid produced and secreted by the ciliary epithelium travels from the posterior chamber around the pupil to the angle where it passes through the specialised multi-layered network of fenestrated lamellae and endothelial cells of the posterior meshwork and into Schlemm's canal. The canal surrounds the posterior meshwork circumferentially (deeper into the ocular tissue) and passes the aqueous into the episcleral venous plexus. The canal of Schlemm is suggested by the pigmented portion of the trabecular meshwork but can only be visualised if blood is refluxed back from the venous system. This will occur if pressure is applied to the eye with a large aperture gonioscope such that the pressure in the draining veins exceeds the intraocular pressure. This can also occur in ocular hypotony and other conditions such as carotid sinus fistula.[2]

4.5.3 SCLERAL SPUR

The scleral spur is a white protrusion of the sclera into the anterior chamber on which rests Schlemm's canal and to which attaches the trabecular meshwork anteriorly and the longitudinal muscle of the ciliary body posteriorly. The spur becomes more visible when the ciliary body and trabeculum are pigmented. Visualisation of the spur verifies that the drainage through the trabeculum is unobstructed in the area being observed.

4.5.4 CILIARY BODY

As with other angle structures, the ciliary body band exhibits extensive variation among individuals. Representing the longitudinal muscle of the ciliary body, the ciliary body band may appear black, brown, gray, or even mottled and mixed with white, and is situated just posterior to the scleral spur. Observation of this band allows a quick determination that the angle is wide open. An excessively wide ciliary body band with a history of trauma may indicate angle recession. **Iris processes** are found in approximately one third of normal eyes and are strands of the uvea which project anteriorly onto the ciliary body or scleral spur and occasionally more anteriorly onto the trabecular meshwork (Fig. 4.6b).

4.5.5 IRIS ROOT

The iris root runs from the last roll of the iris and inserts onto and may obscure the view of the ciliary body.

4.5.6 OTHER GONIOSCOPIC FINDINGS

Pigmentation

Pigmentation is normally present in the angle especially in older patients and those with more pigmented irides, and also in conditions such as pigment dispersion and pseudoexfoliation syndromes (Figs 4.6b and 4.7). Pigment usually deposits most heavily in the inferior quadrant. Trauma and surgery can also cause pigment deposition in the angle.

Peripheral anterior synechiae

Peripheral anterior synechiae (PAS) are abnormal adhesions of the iris to the trabecular meshwork or other angle structures (Fig. 4.8). PAS vary in appearance depending on the aetiology of the adhesion. Angle closure PAS are usually found superiorly where the angle is narrowest whereas inflammatory PAS are more broadly based and are often located inferiorly due to settling of inflammatory debris. Iridocorneal endothelial syndrome often causes severe peripheral anterior synechiae that may advance anteriorly to Schwalbe's line (rare otherwise). PAS due to argon laser trabeculoplasty often appear tooth shaped and can occur if the laser burns are placed too far posteriorly on the pigmented trabeculum or scleral spur.

Iris vessels

Iris vessels from the major arterial circle can be seen as a normal finding in widely open lightly pigmented angles (Fig. 4.6a).

Angle neovascularisation

Neovascularisation in the angle may be preceded by small tufts of rubeosis iridis at the pupillary ruff. The new angle vessels may give the trabeculum a pinkish tone before trunk vessels become visible, bridging the scleral spur.

Angle recession

Blunt trauma may cause posterior displacement and a tear in the ciliary body which manifests as an

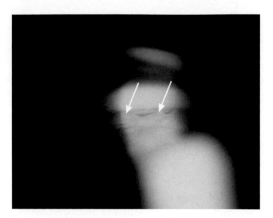

Fig. 4.8 Multiple peripheral anterior synechiae (arrows) in a patient with iridocorneal endothelial (ICE) syndrome.

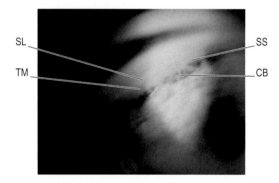

Fig. 4.9 Angle recession following blunt ocular trauma. Note the abnormally wide ciliary body (CB) band in some locations. The trabecular meshwork (TM; greyish band) and Schwalbe's line (SL) are easily distinguished. SS, scleral spur.

angle recession (Fig. 4.9). A widened angle recess (wider ciliary body band) is noted in one or all of the quadrants. Concurrent damage to the trabecular meshwork is the likely cause for the development of angle recession glaucoma. A cyclodialysis cleft, which directs the aqueous into the suprachoroidal space causing hypotony, may also be observed.

4.6 ADDITIONAL EXAMINATION TECHNIQUES

Certain illumination and manipulation techniques can be used to assist the clinician both to diagnos-

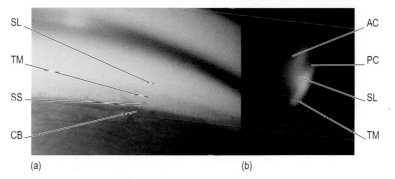

Fig. 4.10 (a) Normal angle. Note the wide mildly pigmented trabecular meshwork (TM) above the narrow white strip of the scleral spur (SS) and band of darker ciliary body (CB). Small flecks of pigment can be seen. Schwalbe's line (SL) is not readily distinguishable. (b) The focal line or slit technique is used to localise Schwalbe's line in narrow and difficult angles. This 'Y' image results from using an optic section, in this case on the right side. The double beam delineates the anterior (AC, left) and posterior (PC, right) surfaces of the cornea. These two come together at the termination of Descemet's membrane (and the cornea) at Schwalbe's line. Below the junction lie the structures of the anterior chamber angle.

tically interpret the gonioscopic view in patients with narrow angles and to therapeutically break an angle closure attack.

4.6.1 FOCAL LINE OR SLIT TECHNIQUE (Fig. 4.10)

The focal line technique is an essential tool for the gonioscopist to master to be able to interpret both narrow and unusual angles. This supplemental technique is used when the angle structures are not unequivocally identifiable by simple inspection.

All of the structures and abnormalities of the angle can be more readily classified if the most anterior angle structure, Schwalbe's line, is first identified. The focal line technique involves projecting a very fine bright optic section at the most oblique angle possible whilst maintaining the section in the mirror of the indirect gonioscope. The corneal section will be observed from the concave surface view and forms a three-dimensional doubled image, much as it is seen in a corneal section in the biomicroscope. The beams of light from the anterior surface will unite or collapse into the posterior surface beam at the termination of the cornea, Schwalbe's line (Fig. 4.10b). The beam will appear to be a two-dimensional (single) line of light from Schwalbe's line posteriorly onto the rest of the angle structures.[5,8] This technique consis-

tently delineates the most anterior angle structure so that significant errors, such as mistaking a pigmented Schwalbe's for the trabecular meshwork, or a pigmented trabeculum for the ciliary body, can be avoided.

4.6.2 TECHNIQUE FOR ANGLE OBSERVATION PAST A CONVEX IRIS

When the view into the angle with a scleral-type lens is obscured by the convexity of the iris, the examiner may facilitate observation over the bowed iris by altering the lens tilt relative to the patient's iris and anterior chamber angle contour. This can be achieved by having the patient look *towards* the mirror (i.e. *away* from the quadrant being viewed) (Fig. 4.11). This allows the anterior plano surface of the lens to be maintained perpendicularly to the viewing axis of the slit lamp, reducing distortions, while at the same time the rays from the deepest part of the angle may get past the forwardly bowed iris. This can also be facilitated by tilting the lens away from the location of the mirror placement. Either way, the clinician should be mindful of the degree of pressure needed to maintain contact of the lens to the cornea and therefore avoid having bubbles introduced in the lens well. This technique is not as useful with corneal-type lenses. However, a slight tilt of the

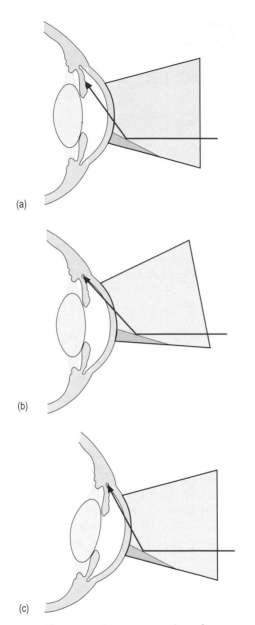

(a)

(b)

(c)

Fig. 4.11 Diagrammatic representation of visualisation over a convex iris with a gonioprism.
Fig. 4.11a and b A corneal lens is represented and is shown in primary position (Fig. 4.11a) and then tilted away from the mirror being used in Fig. 4.11b.
Fig. 4.11c Tilting with a scleral lens is better performed by maintaining the lens in the primary position and having the patient look toward the mirror. This reduces distortion by keeping the flat surface perpendicular to the observation beam.

lens away from the mirror may be used while the patient continues to fixate straight ahead so that contact is maintained.[1,2]

4.6.3 INDENTATION (COMPRESSION) GONIOSCOPY[1]

This technique is invaluable when evaluating a patient with angle closure as it enables a dynamic view of the peripheral iris relative to the trabecular meshwork. It is also used therapeutically to help break a primary pupillary block angle closure attack. Only the corneal-type lenses may be used for this technique; scleral-type lenses merely retro-displace the globe if pressure is applied.

The angle should first be evaluated with gonioscopy and the cornea cleared with hyperosmotic solution if needed. The convex iris and focal line techniques should be used to determine if Schwalbe's line is visible. Note the line of contact of the iris with the angle or posterior cornea. Observe the angle as pressure is applied directly onto the apex of the cornea (Fig. 4.12). As the scleral ring stretches, the peripheral iris and ciliary body will bow backward and aqueous is forced into the angle. If the previously hidden pigmented portion of the trabecular meshwork becomes visible with indentation, appositional angle closure exists (Fig. 4.12b). Synechial angle closure is evident when PAS continue to obscure the angle structures despite the force attempting to open the angle[5,8] (Fig. 4.12c). This usually occurs when the closure has been recurrent, is long-standing and when inflammation has occurred.

4.7 ANGLE CLASSIFICATION SYSTEMS

A number of grading systems have been proposed to attempt to describe the characteristics of the anterior chamber drainage angle.[1-6] However, these systems may insufficiently describe and therefore complicate the characterisation of the angle because they are either not fully descriptive or vary from one system to the next. For instance, the same label for a wide open angle from one grading system may represent a very narrow angle in another.

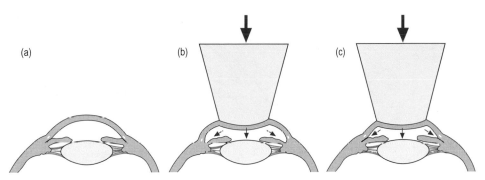

Fig. 4.12a   Eye showing angle closure.

Fig. 4.12b   Indentation or compression gonioscopy. A corneal lens is used to compress the cornea centrally in an eye with angle closure to attempt to break the attack and differentiate appositional versus synechial angle closure. Appositional closure exists if the previously hidden trabecular meshwork becomes visible with indentation.

Fig. 4.12c   An angle with synechial closure remains closed despite compression.

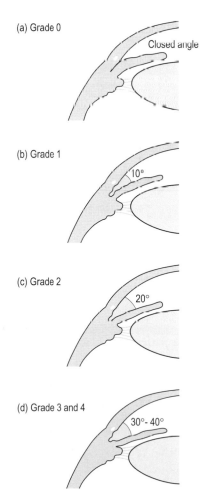

(a) Grade 0

Closed angle

(b) Grade 1

10°

(c) Grade 2

20°

(d) Grade 3 and 4

30°- 40°

The **Shaffer** system (Fig. 4.13) grades the angle by the estimate of the geometrical angle between the iris and angle wall at the recess. This system most closely correlates with the van Herick angle estimation method where the shadow created by an optical section directed at the lateral (nasal and temporal) limbus is compared to the width of the optic section. Angles grade 3–4 are widely open; that is, the angle depth is one half to one full thickness of the corneal section for a 30–40° approach. In both the van Herick and Shaffer systems, angles designated grade 2 or less are considered *capable* of closure: angle depth of one quarter the optical section and angular approach of 20°, respectively. Angles designated grade 0 are considered closed.

Spaeth expanded the above grading (Fig. 4.14) to include important information such as the peripheral iris contour (regular, steep or queer) and the site of iris insertion (anterior to Schwalbe's line to the ciliary body). Characterisation of all three parts of the Spaeth system are important in

Fig. 4.13a–d   Representation of Shaffer grading system demonstrating characterisation by angular approach only. Grade 4 = 40° or more, grade 3 = 30°, grade 2 = 20°, grade 1 = ~10°, slit-like = open only a few degrees, and grade 0 = closed. No designation is given for the contour of the iris or the location of iris insertion.

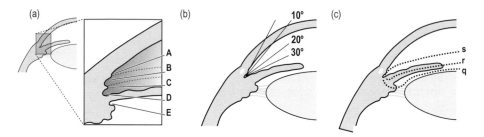

Fig. 4.14a–c Representation of Spaeth grading system. Three criteria are used to describe the angle: (a) the point of insertion on the angle wall (*A* is anterior to SL, *B* is behind SL, *C* is at the SS, *D* is a deep angle with CB visible, and *E* is extremely deep). The iris is shown in an arbitrary position in the figure, but could be as anterior as A or as posterior as E, (b) the angular approach in degrees of the iris at the angle recess, and (c) the configuration of the most peripheral portion of the iris (*r* for regular, *s* for steep, and *q* for queer indicating a concave configuration). Therefore C30r represents an angle open to the scleral spur with a regular configuration to the iris and a 30° approach at the angle recess. Adapted with permission from Kanski J. Clinical Ophthalmology, 3rd edn. Oxford: Butterworth-Heinemann, 1994.

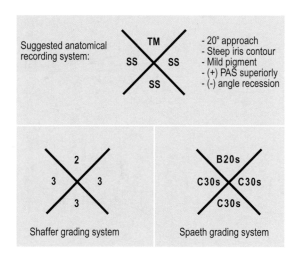

Fig. 4.15 An example of a recording of the suggested anatomical grading system. Comparison is made with the Shaffer and Spaeth systems. Each demonstrates examination in all four quadrants.

determining a patient's risk of both angle closure and other glaucomas.

4.8 SUGGESTED ANATOMICAL RECORDING SYSTEM

Determining the relative openness of an angle is the most common reason for using a gonioscope. However, the anatomy and appearance of the angle vary greatly between individuals and should be accurately recorded. To eliminate the problems of difficult categorisation and the discrepancies between grading systems, it is suggested that the clinician record the angle information in a descriptive way without using a number grade.

Anatomically the anterior chamber angle is widest inferiorly, then temporally, nasally, and is narrowest superiorly.[3] All quadrants should be inspected, preferably in a continuous manner, by following the mirror through 360° of rotation. It is recommended that the inferior angle be examined first as the structures are most easily identified in the widest angle with the most pigment.

The angle should be carefully evaluated and documentation should always include: 1) the most posterior structure seen (location of iris insertion), 2) the approach of the angle at the recess (in degrees) and the contour of the iris, as well as 3) the amount of pigment, and the presence of iris processes, angle recession, peripheral anterior synechiae, and normal and abnormal vasculature (Fig. 4.15).

4.9 SUMMARY

Gonioscopy is the standard procedure for examination of the anterior chamber angle and is a critical technique in primary eye care. The clinician must practise the technique and observe many angles as enormous variation can be noted in both normal and abnormal angles by the experienced observer. Gonioscopy is essential to master not only for the assessment of a patient's risk for angle closure with dilation, but also in the diagnosis and subsequent management of the open and closed angle glaucomas and many other anterior segment anomalies.

Acknowledgements
Thanks to Anne Weber for illustrations.

Disclaimer: The authors have no proprietary interest in the equipment outlined in this article.

References

1. Prokopich CL, Flanagan JG. Gonioscopy: evaluation of the anterior chamber angle. Part I. Ophthal Physiol Opt 1996; 16:s39–42.
2. Fisch BM. Gonioscopy and the Glaucomas. Boston: Butterworth-Heinemann; 1993.
3. Ritch R, Shields MB, Krupin T. The Glaucomas. St. Louis: CV Mosby Company; 1989.
4. Shields MB. Textbook of Glaucoma, 3rd edn. Baltimore: Williams & Wilkins; 1992.
5. Kanski JJ, McAllister JA. Glaucoma: A Colour Manual of Diagnosis and Treatment. Oxford: Butterworth-Heinemann Ltd; 1989.
6. Lewis TL, Fingeret M. Primary Care of the Glaucomas. Norwalk: Appleton & Lange; 1993.
7. van Herick W, Shaffer RN, Schwartz A. Estimation of the width of angle of anterior chamber. Incidence and significance of the narrow angle. Am J Ophthalmol 1969; 68:626–629.
8. Van Buskirk EM. Clinical Atlas of Glaucoma. Philadelphia: WB Saunders Company; 1986.
9. Gorin G, Posner A. Slit-Lamp Gonioscopy. Baltimore: Williams & Wilkins Company; 1967.
10. Alward WLM. Color Atlas of Gonioscopy. Barcelona: Wolfe; 1994.
11. Woodard DR, Woodard RB. Handbook of Drugs in Primary Eyecare. Norwalk: Appleton & Lange; 1991.

Chapter 5

Interpretation of visual field measures from automated and semi-automated perimeters

Alicja R Rudnicka and David F Edgar

CHAPTER CONTENTS

5.1 INTRODUCTION

This chapter describes some of the testing algorithms for the measurement and interpretation of visual function that are most likely to be used in glaucoma management. Although this chapter concentrates on the Henson and Humphrey Field Analyzer ranges of instruments the fundamental principles are transferable to other semi-automated or automated perimeters.

5.2 RETINAL LIGHT SENSITIVITY AND THE DECIBEL

Many perimeters record visual light sensitivity in terms of the decibel (dB), which is a measure of retinal light sensitivity. In relative terms, a higher dB value means that the retina is more sensitive and the differential light threshold value would be lower, i.e. a dimmer light intensity value. Photometric units (such as apostilbs (asb)) may be used to specify the luminance of the stimulus, but visual field plots are usually labelled in decibels. Most instruments display a key showing the relationship between apostilbs and decibels. Changes in light intensity can be achieved by the use of neutral density filters, which are calibrated in log units of optical density. A neutral density filter of 1.0 reduces the light intensity by a factor of 10; a filter of 2.0 reduces the light intensity by a factor of 100 and so on. A change on the decibel scale of 1.0 dB is equivalent to a 0.1 unit change in log units. The actual light intensity level that is recorded by a perimeter is unique to that particular instrument, so the absolute values are not directly comparable across different makes of perimeter because the scale created by the manufacturers is relative.

Visual field testing gives a direct measure of visual function that is non-invasive, but despite advances in the automation of perimetry the subjective nature of the test remains, since it depends upon the patient's subjective responses. There are three important physiological factors that should be considered in connection with automated or semi-automated perimetry, namely learning, fatigue and within-patient fluctuations in retinal light sensitivity, and these are not necessarily mutually exclusive.

5.3 LEARNING AND FATIGUE

The presence of a learning process with subjects new to automated perimetry is well established.[1-3] It is usually demonstrated as an improvement in the mean sensitivity, mean deviation, and both short- and long-term fluctuations (see section 5.4). Consequently, one baseline visual field test is insufficient, as a later reduction in the field may not be detected because the learning process counterbalances the true loss in sensitivity, and these two effects may cancel each other out. A number of investigators believe most of the learning to be complete after the performance of the first or second field tests. However, learning has been shown to continue beyond the first two field tests in some subjects, particularly if their baseline sensitivity values are low.[3-6] In general, it is good practice to allow at least one training visual field test per eye to account for learning effects.

The effort and attention required for automated perimetry may adversely influence the sensitivity and reliability of the field test results. An increase in the threshold with increasing test duration has been demonstrated with automated perimetry. These fatigue effects, which tend to increase with examination duration and which are greatest in or adjacent to relative scotomata, have been reported in glaucoma.[7-12] This is not surprising since the assessment of defective fields tends to take longer than the assessment of 'normal' fields because more questions need to be asked by the perimeter in order to plot these defects. This may explain, to some extent, the enhancement or exaggeration of visual field defects with automated perimetry as compared with manual perimetry. With the advent of faster testing strategies, such as the Swedish Interactive Threshold Algorithm (SITA) (see below), the problems associated with fatigue are reduced.

5.4 WITHIN-PATIENT FLUCTUATIONS IN RETINAL LIGHT SENSITIVITY

If the visual threshold is measured several times at a location the result is not always identical. This variability of the threshold has been termed fluctuation, and is divided into a short-term and a long-term component. Short-term fluctuation (SF) is the variation within a single examination. It depends largely on the uncertain responses for stimuli near threshold, which is described by the frequency-of-seeing curve (see Chapter 7). The amount of fluctuation is influenced by the visual sensitivity, patient reliability and the strategy employed by the instrument. SF has been shown to be greatest in the superior field and to increase with increasing eccentricity, especially for eccentricities beyond 30°.[12-16] It is now accepted that an early indication of visual field loss may be an increase in the localised fluctuation (see Chapter 7). Long-term fluctuation is an additional component of the variability encountered when tests are performed on separate occasions. Long-term fluctuation decreases with perimetric learning.[5,12]

5.5 PATTERNS OF VISUAL FIELD LOSS IN GLAUCOMA

The distribution and arrangement of the retinal nerve fibres govern the pattern of visual field loss in glaucoma. The retinal nerve fibres from the retina temporal to the fovea arch above and below the macula to enter the optic disc, and they congregate at the upper and lower poles of the disc. The fibres from the temporal retina are usually most susceptible to damage in primary open

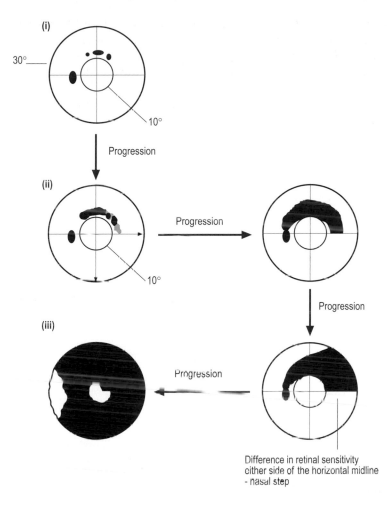

Fig. 5.1   Patterns of visual field loss in open angle glaucoma:
(i) isolated paracentral scotomata following the course of retinal nerve fibre bundles,

(ii) paracentral scotomata coalesce to form an arcuate defect, and

(iii) arcuate defects break through to periphery. In advanced cases only the macular area is spared, possibly together with a small island in the temporal periphery. In extreme cases there is complete loss of visual function over the entire field.

angle glaucoma (POAG). The nerve fibres from the temporal retina do not cross the midline (horizontal raphé) and scotomata follow the shape of these nerve fibre bundles, giving rise to characteristic glaucomatous field defects which may be absolute, or relative, or a combination of both (Fig. 5.1) comprising:

- Isolated paracentral scotomata at 10–20° eccentricity (usually the upper field is affected initially), which may be relative (as shown by gray areas in Fig. 5.1) or absolute defects.
- Paracentral scotomata can increase in number and expand or coalesce to form arcuate defects.
- Scotomata can extend in an arcuate shape from the upper or lower poles of the blind spot.
- Nasal step – resulting from asymmetry in retinal sensitivity either side of the temporal horizontal midline because these nerve fibres do not cross

the horizontal midline. This sign is highly specific to POAG.

As the disease progresses the arcuate defects extend to the blind spot, and they may also widen and break through to the periphery and expand centrally. In advanced stages of glaucoma a central 2–3° island of vision may remain, possibly accompanied by an area of field in the temporal periphery. In extreme cases there is complete loss of visual function over the entire field.

Given that the temporal retinal nerve fibres do not cross the horizontal midline, it is not unusual for one hemisphere to be more affected than the other, and the corresponding field defects do not cross the horizontal midline. More commonly the upper hemifield is preferentially affected. In more advanced cases both hemispheres become involved but the asymmetry between upper and lower fields usually remains. Although POAG is a bilateral condition, its progression is often asymmetrical, with one eye affected to a greater extent than the other, leading to asymmetrical visual field defects.

Arcuate defects can also occur with chorioretinal lesions that follow an arcuate shape (such as myopic degeneration), branch vein occlusion, branch artery occlusion or atypical retinitis pigmentosa. Papilloedema, drusen of the optic disc, papillitis, anterior ischaemic optic neuropathy, and retrobulbar neuritis can also give rise to arcuate field defects.

Baring of the blind spot is no longer regarded as a typical field defect in glaucoma because it can be reproduced in patients without ocular disease. It can occur as an artefact of kinetic perimetry associated with a physiological phenomenon arising from the fact that the inferior retina is less sensitive than the superior, and when isopters near threshold are plotted using kinetic perimetry the isopter plot may border the blind spot, i.e. baring of the blind spot. However, it can occur as an extension of an arcuate defect, but baring of the blind spot itself is not specific to POAG. Similarly enlargement of the blind spot can occur as part of an extending arcuate defect, but enlargement of the blind spot can also occur in many different pathologies.

Diffuse or generalised depression of the field may occur as a result of diffuse loss to the nerve fibres, but this is a non-specific sign in glaucoma and can occur in many diseases affecting visual function, such as opacification of the crystalline lens. Depression of the field may also result from small pupils, incorrect correction of refractive error and patient fatigue.

5.6 THE HENSON RANGE OF INSTRUMENTS

Early models of the Henson perimeters (e.g. Henson CFA 3000/3200 and CFS 2000; Tinsley Medical Instruments, Croydon, England) use LED stimuli that subtend approximately 0.5° at the patient's eye. The LEDs have flat diffusing front surfaces 3.0 mm in diameter that are mounted flush within a flat gray screen. The reflec-

tive properties of the screen have been matched to those of the LEDs, when not activated, to minimise the possibility of the patient being aware of any black hole effects. The LEDs have a broad spectral output (530–600 nm) with a maximum intensity of $300 \, cd/m^2$, and a stimulus presentation time of 200 ms.

The patient is seated approximately 33 cm from the screen, allowing the central 25° of the visual field to be investigated. For these early models the background luminance of the test is $0.25 \, cd/m^2$. Multiple stimulus suprathreshold testing (semi-automated) is available on all models, and single stimulus full-threshold testing (fully-automated) is available on the CFA 3200 and 3000.[17]

5.6.1 SUPRATHRESHOLD MULTIPLE STIMULUS STRATEGIES FOR CFS 2000 AND CFA 3000/3200

Determination of the test threshold, which in turn determines the initial intensity at which the suprathreshold test is carried out, is a key step if any suprathreshold perimetry test is to be performed efficiently. If the initial intensity at which the suprathreshold test is carried out is set at too high a level (initial presentation of stimuli too bright) this will lead to field defects being missed and will reduce the sensitivity of the test. Setting the initial intensity too low (initial presentation of stimuli too dim) leads to an overestimate of field defects, will reduce the specificity of the test and will lead to too many false positives.[18] Such is the importance of threshold determination in suprathreshold testing that the method to be used may be stipulated in the protocol for a glaucoma co-managed care scheme. In the early Henson instruments the test threshold is established manually using a selection of test patterns and the recommended method of manual threshold estimation makes use of a 'seen to non-seen' approach:

- Initially present a stimulus at a light intensity that is easy for the patient to see.
- Reduce the light intensity in 1 dB (or 0.1 log unit) steps until no stimulus is seen.
- Confirm no stimulus is seen using another pattern.
- Threshold is 1 dB brighter than this.
- Use a different pattern at each presentation.

This method of manually determining threshold gives reasonable performance compared with the more accurate but clinically impractical method of manually finding the threshold at each location.[18] The 'seen to non-seen' approach described above takes about 30 seconds per eye. It is the preferred approach if a field defect is present, rather than the alternative 'non-seen to seen' method. Patients prefer the 'seen to non-seen' approach, which builds patient confidence, and it serves a useful training role for the suprathreshold testing which follows the threshold determination. The automated determination of threshold has been incorporated into later Henson models (see below).

Once the threshold has been determined, the suprathreshold strategies initially start testing at an intensity 5 dB (0.5 log units) brighter than the threshold estimate. Three levels of investigation are available, related to the number of locations that can be tested. These are:

- 26 retinal locations (designed for screening).
- 68 retinal locations (designed for patients where a field defect is suspected or there are other reasons for performing a more rigorous test).
- 136 retinal locations (designed to establish the extent of a defect).

In glaucoma co-managed care schemes the level of the test will almost certainly be specified in the protocol and is likely to be the 136 location test, which is most appropriate for monitoring stable glaucoma. Locations that are missed at 5 dB brighter than threshold can be retested at 8 dB and 12 dB brighter than threshold. At the end of the testing procedure a score is produced by the instrument, which indicates the likelihood that the current field comes from a patient with a normal, suspicious or defective field.[17]

5.6.2 FULL-THRESHOLD STRATEGY FOR CFA 3000/3200

The single stimulus full-threshold programme tests 52 locations within the central 25° using a fully automated procedure. The patient is required to respond to each seen presentation by pressing a button. The algorithm adopted by the machine is a repetitive bracketing procedure with step sizes of 4 dB reducing to 2 dB after the first reversal. Catch trials are also incorporated to estimate the false-positive and false-negative rates, and the final results are analysed to give a series of indices. These are mean defect, loss variance, corrected loss variance and fluctuation (these indices are essentially equivalent to those of the Humphrey Field Analyzer, and are described later in this chapter).

5.6.3 HENSON PRO RANGE

The Henson range of instruments has evolved over the years and currently available models include the Henson Pro Compact 6000, and the Henson Pro 3500 and 5000. These comprise a 25 cm radius bowl perimeter, which extends visual field testing to an eccentricity of 72° into the periphery of the visual field, and these perimeters have full-threshold and suprathreshold strategies which are fully automated. High intensity green LED stimuli, with a broad spectral output ranging from 540 nm to 590 nm, project onto the smooth back surface of the translucent bowl, with the result that nothing is visible to the patient until the LED is activated (i.e. no black hole effects). The stimuli have a 18 dB (1.8 log units) range of stimulus intensity up to a maximum of 1000 cd/m^2. The background luminance is 3.15 cd/m^2 (10 asb). Stimuli have an angular subtense of 0.5°, equivalent to a Goldmann III stimulus, and the stimulus presentation time is 200 ms. The Henson Pro Range contains a range of programmes using full-threshold methods covering the peripheral, central and macular regions of the field.[17]

5.6.4 THE HEART ALGORITHM

For suprathreshold perimetry the threshold determination has been automated using the HEART algorithm. The new algorithm begins by selecting an intensity 1 dB brighter than the mean age threshold value for the patient. It determines the threshold at each of four key locations using a single fixed step size of 1 dB and six presentations at each location. These locations are symmetrically situated, one in each quadrant, 12.7° from fixation along the 45°, 135°, 225° and 315° meridians.[19] For most patients, the data from the last four presentations at these four locations are averaged to give the final threshold estimate. There are

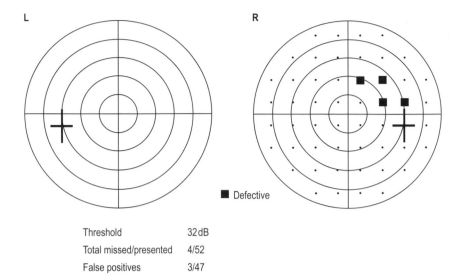

Threshold	32 dB
Total missed/presented	4/52
False positives	3/47

Fig. 5.2 Early arcuate glaucomatous defect in the patient's right eye, plotted using suprathreshold methods, on the Henson Pro 5000. The HEART algorithm was used to establish the initial threshold estimate, together with the multisampling programme which employs a 3/5 pass/fail criterion at each location tested. The multisampling programme tests 52 locations within the central 24°, and uses a single intensity setting of 5 dB brighter than threshold.

precautions built into the algorithm to guard against the effects of widespread field loss affecting the determination of the threshold.

5.6.5 MULTISAMPLING

In conventional suprathreshold perimetry each stimulus location is tested on a maximum of two occasions. If the stimulus is seen at the first presentation, that location is assumed to have no significant field defect and no further testing is carried out. If the stimulus is not seen at the first presentation, to guard against a false negative response, a second presentation is made. If the second presentation is seen, the location is assumed to have no significant field defect. If the second presentation is not seen, the location is assumed to be defective, and may be investigated in more detail. This approach, often referred to as '1/2 pass/fail criterion', is justifiable in general optometric practice where the prevalence of significant visual field defects is low. It gives high specificity at the price of lowered sensitivity. Henson and Artes[19] noted that in high-risk patients and for the monitoring of patients with known visual field loss, precisely the types of patient monitored by optometrists in co-managed care schemes, a test procedure which has a higher sensitivity is required. They have devised a multisampling approach to the determination of the initial threshold which has been incorporated into the Henson Pro 5000 instrument. Multisampling uses a 3/5 pass/fail criterion rather than the conventional 1/2 criterion. The minimum number of presentations at each location is 3, with a maximum of 5. If the suprathreshold stimulus is seen three times at a location, no significant field defect is assumed to exist. If the suprathreshold stimulus is missed three times at a location, then the location is assumed to be defective. Added advantages of multisampling, as tested in simulated visual fields, are that it gives a more accurate representation of the visual field loss and it gives reduced variability compared with conventional suprathreshold and full-threshold perimetry.[19] Multisampling takes longer than conventional suprathreshold testing but in simulated fields it is roughly equivalent in duration to SITA standard testing. Typical glaucomatous field plots using the HEART algorithm with the multisampling programme are shown in Figs 5.2 and 5.3. The multisampling programme tests 52 locations within the central 24°, and uses a single intensity setting of 5 dB brighter than threshold.

5.7 THE HUMPHREY FIELD ANALYZER

The Humphrey Field Analyzer (HFA) range of instruments (Humphrey Instruments, California USA) are automated computer-driven projection

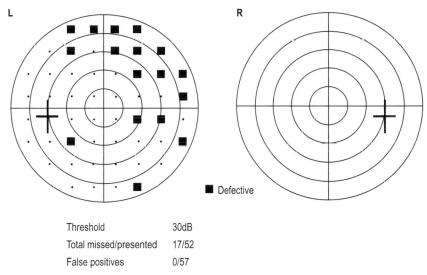

Fig. 5.3 Moderate arcuate glaucomatous defects in the patient's left eye affecting both superior and inferior hemifields, plotted using suprathreshold methods on the Henson Pro 5000 perimeter. The inferior defect demonstrates a nasal step. The HEART algorithm was used to establish the initial threshold estimate, together with the multisampling programme which employs a 3/5 pass/fail criterion. The multisampling programme tests 52 locations within the central 24°, and uses a single intensity setting of 5 dB brighter than threshold.

perimeters providing a choice of threshold and suprathreshold programmes. The testing procedure is fully automated and visual field test results can be printed or stored on computer for future reference. The stimulus parameters and bowl dimensions were originally based on the Goldmann bowl perimeter. The HFA projects a single stimulus onto a hemispherical surface by the use of mirrors which are operated by a motor. The background luminance is fixed at 31.5 asb (10 cd/m²) while stimulus luminance can be varied over a 5.1 log unit range (0.08–10 000 asb) through a set of neutral density filters plus a filter wedge. The decibel is the unit of retinal sensitivity on the HFA. In the HFA:

$$\text{Retinal sensitivity in dB} = 10 \log(L_b/\Delta L) + 25$$

where L_b is background luminance, and ΔL is the stimulus luminance.

Stimulus positioning is automatically checked and adjusted at the beginning of each test. Edge detectors recheck correct mirror positioning each time the mirror passes the positions corresponding to the vertical and horizontal meridians of the visual field. The order of presentation of stimuli is random and the entire testing procedure is auto-

mated by recording the patient's response to each presentation, which is to press a button if they see a light stimulus.

The HFA has become the instrument of choice in many institutions, with programmes 24-2 (54 locations within 24° of fixation) or 30-2 (76 locations in the central 30°) being used as standard (Table 5.1). In these programmes the stimuli are arranged either side of the midlines and are separated by 6° (Figs. 5.5–5.10 illustrate the 24-2 programme). Additional features include:

- An eye video monitor which enables the patient's eye to be viewed during testing and aids positioning the patient's pupil at the centre of the hemisphere.
- Gaze tracking systems to monitor fixation.
- Kinetic perimetry.

5.7.1 SUPRATHRESHOLD SCREENING STRATEGIES

Age reference screening strategy

The patient's date of birth is entered into the machine prior to testing. For the screening test

Table 5.1   **Technical specifications of the Humphrey Field Analyzer**

Stimulus	Mode of presentation	Static and random
Specifications	Duration	0.2 seconds
	Source	Incandescent lamp
	Intensities	0.08–10 000 apostilbs
	Intensity range	5.1 log units
	Size	0.25–64 mm²
	Colours	White, blue, red
Background	Surface shape	Hemisphere, 30/33 cm radius
	Luminance	31.5 asb

the stimulus intensity is set to 6 dB brighter than the expected threshold level for a given age, and the results are compared with age matched 'normal' data stored in the perimeter. Any locations not seen on retesting are recorded as defects.

Threshold related screening strategy

A 'normal' field contour is constructed for each eye by the HFA using the second-most sensitive threshold value of four primary locations (one in each quadrant). This reference hill of vision is automatically corrected for both the patient's age and the decline in retinal sensitivity with eccentricity. The instrument determines a value known as the 'central reference level', which is recorded and stored and appears on the printout so that the brightness level at which the test was run is known. Stimulus intensity is set to 6 dB brighter than the threshold expected at each location from the reference hill of vision that has been constructed. Any locations missed on a first presentation and not seen on retesting are recorded as defects.

Age reference and threshold related screening categorise locations into either seen or missed twice at the screening level. Alternative screening strategies are available which provide more information on the missed locations:

1. Three zone screening strategy

Locations that are missed twice at the screening level are retested using the brightest stimulus available (10 000 asb). Locations seen at this level are

therefore relative defects and those missed at this level are classified as absolute defects. Three outcomes are possible at each location on the field plot:

- seen at screening level
- missed at screening level, but seen at 10 000 asb (relative defect)
- missed at screening level and not seen at 10 000 asb (absolute defect).

2. Quantify defect

Locations that are missed twice at screening level are thresholded (the threshold algorithm is described below).

5.7.2 THRESHOLD STRATEGIES

Full-threshold

The 'up and down staircase method', utilised by the HFA was, until recently, the most commonly used threshold testing strategy (see SITA strategy below). To obtain threshold the light intensity level descends/ascends by 4 dB until the first reversal (from seen to not seen or vice versa), and then ascends/descends by 2 dB staircase until the second reversal. The last seen value is recorded as threshold. This is called the 4-2 dB staircase algorithm since the stimulus intensity is altered first in 4 dB (0.4 log units) steps then 2 dB (0.2 log units) steps (Fig. 5.4).

At the beginning of a full threshold test, one primary location in each quadrant is tested twice,

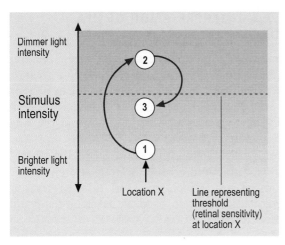

Fig. 5.4 Staircase algorithm: The first stimulus presentation, ①, is at a stimulus intensity brighter than threshold. The second stimulus presentation, ②, is set 4 dB dimmer and this stimulus intensity is dimmer than threshold (first crossing of threshold). The third stimulus presentation, ③, is set 2 dB brighter than that at ② and is just brighter than threshold (second crossing of threshold). At many locations five or more presentations may be required because the initial presentation may be considerably brighter (or dimmer) than threshold.

$(x = \pm 9°$ and $y = \pm 9°)$ see Fig. 5.5. These four seed locations are used as starting levels for establishing threshold for neighbouring locations, which are assumed to drop by 0.3 dB for each degree of eccentricity. Results from secondary locations are then used as starting levels (adjusted for eccentricity) for their neighbouring locations and so on. If the measured threshold at a location differs by more than a certain amount from the expected value (which is based on the threshold of the neighbouring location) the threshold is measured again. Stimuli are presented randomly, which has been found to improve the stability of patients' fixation, probably because the stimulus duration is too short for the patient to benefit from directing their attention to it, unlike with manual kinetic perimetry.

Full threshold testing of, for example, 76 locations within the central 30° takes about 15 minutes per eye. To shorten testing times various other algorithms have been introduced, namely full-threshold from prior data, Fast threshold, FASTPAC and SITA. Of these, SITA offers the greatest time saving with performance that may be as good as full-threshold, and SITA has become the testing strategy of choice.

Other threshold strategies utilising the 4-2 dB algorithm include the following.

Full-threshold from prior data

Performs the standard 4-2 dB staircase algorithm but utilises the patient's previous results as the starting point.

Fast threshold

Stimuli are presented at each location 2 dB brighter than the threshold recorded at the previous test, with only missed locations thresholded.

FASTPAC

This algorithm uses a single 3 dB crossing of threshold instead of the 4-2 dB approach. Examination time is reduced by approximately one third. A 76-point central 30° programme takes about 9 minutes. However, FASTPAC is less accurate than the 4-2 dB procedure.

Swedish interactive threshold algorithm

The introduction of SITA was an important step towards considerably reducing testing times.[20] There are two SITA algorithms available, SITA Standard and SITA Fast. The SITA Standard strategy takes roughly half the time of the conventional 4-2 dB staircase algorithm, and SITA Fast takes roughly half the time of FASTPAC. The time required to test 76 locations within the central 30° is about 6–8 minutes with SITA standard and 3–4 minutes with SITA Fast.[21] SITA standard is believed to offer improved accuracy and reproducibility compared with the 4-2 dB algorithm and SITA Fast is comparable to FASTPAC.[22–27]

The SITA method of obtaining threshold at each location utilises information obtained throughout the field test to continually update the testing procedure. All available information on the patient's responses during a test is used to refine the final threshold value at all test locations.

SITA testing strategy

- Choice of stimulus brightness is initially based on the age-corrected threshold values of the hill of vision.
- Estimates from neighbouring locations (especially those in the same hemifield) interact to produce a constantly updated hill of vision for the patient.
- Estimates of sensitivity at any given stimulus location are determined based on knowledge of the frequency of seeing curve, the pattern in which glaucomatous visual field defects occur, and how the thresholds at neighbouring locations in the field are related to each other.

Bayesian statistical methods are used to determine when sufficient information has been obtained at each location. The method is underpinned by an estimate of the 'permitted' error in obtaining threshold at a location. If the threshold estimate falls within the accepted limits of error for that location the testing is terminated for that location. Thus more time is spent on locations that require more information. Once the testing has been completed at each location, all information collected during the examination is used to refine the final threshold estimates.

Because stimuli are presented at or near threshold for each location this greatly reduces the number of stimulus presentations required and hence the time taken to complete the test. Additionally, the patient's response times are monitored so that inter-stimulus duration can be adjusted. Reliability of the patient is measured using procedures that differ from older algorithms (see section 5.7.3). SITA defines a false-positive response when the response time falls outside the response time window that has been estimated for the patient. Utilization of response times again reduces testing time because false-positive catch trials are not performed. False negatives are estimated by identifying responses that should have been visible to the patient, based on knowledge of the final determined threshold value.

5.7.3 INTERPRETATION OF HFA FIELDS (FIG. 5.5)

Traditionally, perimetric data has been presented graphically. With automated perimetry a great deal of numerical data is generated and it can be represented in a variety of ways. STATPAC is the statistical analysis package for the HFA and the single field analysis printout of STATPAC is most commonly used. With every printout the date, patient name, programme used, testing strategy, conditions of test, which eye, and time of test (and optionally refraction used, visual acuity and pupil size) can be recorded.

Reliability parameters

These appear near the top left-hand corner of the printout. A patient's responses can be affected by factors such as mood, attention, nervousness, age and cooperation. The reliability indices are an attempt to measure the patient's performance and give an indication of the reliability of the visual field.

At the beginning of every test the position of the patient's blind spot is assumed to be in the average anatomical position. If the blind spot is not in its usual position it is re-plotted. Subsequently, if the patient responds to a supraliminal stimulus projected into the blind spot a **fixation loss** error is recorded. However, a distinction is not possible between a fixation loss (FL) and a **false-positive** (FP) error. An FP error occurs when the patient responds in the absence of a stimulus presentation. At random intervals a suprathreshold stimulus is presented in an area already tested (9 dB brighter than previous response). If the patient fails to respond to this stimulus a **false-negative** (FN) error is recorded. All three of these measures require extra stimuli to be presented so that they can be estimated. Field tests are flagged as unreliable if FL > 20% or if FP or FN > 33%. The HFA prints an 'XX' after any of the reliability indices that fall outside established limits for reliability.

In Fig. 5.5, FL = 0/21; this means that the patient did not respond to any of the 21 supraliminal presentations in the blind spot. This can be interpreted as the patient maintaining steady fixation throughout the test. Also, this patient did not

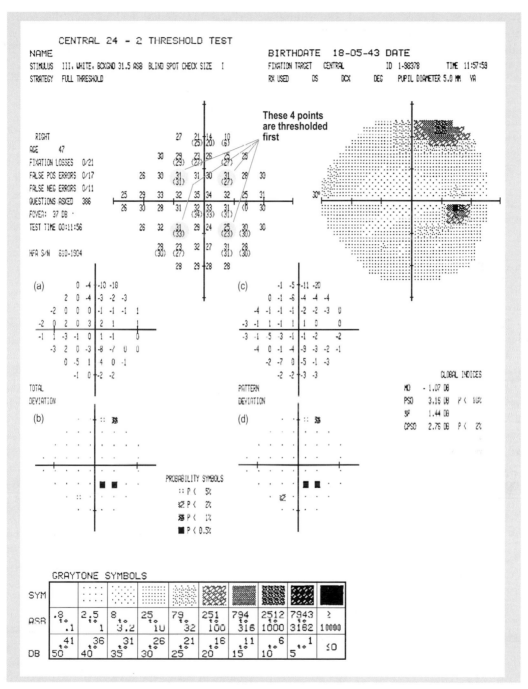

Fig. 5.5 Single field analysis printout from a glaucomatous patient's right eye using a full threshold strategy with the 24-2 programme on the HFA.

have any FP or FN errors. In total 386 stimuli presentations were made. The foveal threshold was 37 dB and the entire test took 11 minutes and 56 seconds.

Numeric plot

The top left numeric plot of the field displays the actual threshold sensitivities in decibel (dB) units. Any locations that are thresholded a second time have thresholds that appear in parenthesis below the original threshold estimate. This format can be difficult to interpret.

Gray scale plot

To the right of the numeric plot is the gray scale plot. Sensitivity values are represented by a gray symbol. Ten gray levels are available, and a key is printed at the bottom of the field printout. Interpolated sensitivities are derived from measured sensitivities at neighbouring locations, and are only slightly less accurate than direct measurements when the inter-stimulus separation does not exceed 6°. However, it has been shown that this form of data presentation can be inaccurate depending upon the interpolation procedure employed. At a glance, gray scales appear easy to interpret but they do not convey other important information.

STATPAC

STATPAC is the statistical package available with the HFA for threshold test results. It encompasses various forms of data presentation, summary statistics for serial visual fields and for global indices. Those from the single field analysis printout are described below. (For other statistical analyses for detecting change see Chapter 7).

Total deviation plots

A field contour is constructed by the HFA and is called the age corrected 'normal' reference field (also referred to as the age matched field). It is determined using the second-most sensitive threshold value of the four primary locations (one in each quadrant), and the patient's age. The dif-

ferences in threshold values from this *reference* field and that measured for a given patient are displayed in two formats, numeric and gray scale. The upper plot (Fig. 5.5a) displays numerical values that represent the difference in decibels between the measured field and that of the age corrected 'normal' threshold values at each location.

In Fig. 5.5 most of the values are within 1 or 2 dB of that expected, but there are a few locations differing by more than 5 dB. These values are converted into gray scale symbols in the lower plot ('b' in Fig. 5.5). In the lower hemifield there are two locations (in the typical arcuate area) with the darkest gray scale symbols (differing by 8 dB and 7 dB from the reference field in the numeric plot).

A key is given to the right of the lower plot, labelled 'probability symbols'. The probability significance levels are 5%, 2%, 1%, and 0.5%. In Fig. 5.5 two locations in the lower hemifield have a probability of <0.5%. This means that less than 0.5% of the 'normal' population are likely to deviate from the reference field by the value found at that location. It is not the probability of being 'abnormal' but gives an indication of how likely the observed difference is in a 'normal' field. In this instance, a probability symbol of <0.5% means that this observation in a 'normal' population is not very likely, less than 1 chance in 200. The locations at the top of the field differ from the 'normal' reference field by a greater amount in absolute terms (10 dB and 18 dB) but have a higher likelihood of occurring in 'normal' fields (p values are less than 5% and 2%). This is because defects at the periphery of the field are commonly associated with drooping lids or lens/frame artefacts and are therefore more likely to be observed in 'normal' fields.

Pattern deviation plots

These are similar to the total deviation plots, except STATPAC has adjusted the test results for any change in the overall height of the hill of vision ('c' in Fig. 5.5). This is in an attempt to separate diffuse from localised changes. For example, if the total deviation plot shows many darker symbols which are less frequent in the corresponding pattern deviation plot, this indicates that the field loss is mainly due to a general reduction in sensitivity with few localised defects. In Fig. 5.5c the two locations in the lower hemifield still remain identified, now differing by

9 dB from the reference field and have a low probability (<0.5%) of being observed in a 'normal' population (Fig. 5.5d). This also tells us that the defect is localised and another location in the lower hemifield has become more prominent in the pattern deviation plot. The pattern of these three locations strongly suggests an arcuate defect.

Global indices

Finally, a short list labelled 'global indices' appears on the far right. Alongside the global indices a probability value may be printed. Once again, these probability values estimate the likelihood of observing a value at least that high or extreme in a 'normal' population.

Mean deviation

Mean deviation (MD) is a weighted average deviation of the measured field from the 'normal' reference field. It is the arithmetic mean of the differences between measured values and 'normal' age-corrected reference field values at the tested locations weighted by the between-subject variability in thresholds. A deviation at a central location where the 'normal' between-subject variability is low carries more weight than the same deviation at a more peripheral location where the 'normal' inter-subject variability is higher. MD estimates the uniform part of the deviation of the measured field from the age-corrected 'normal' reference field. With increasing field defects MD becomes an increasing negative number. In Fig. 5.5 the MD is -1.07 dB, and this patient's field is on average 1.07 dB less sensitive than the age corrected 'normal' reference field. In other words it is 'on average' quite similar to the reference field.

Pattern standard deviation

To determine pattern standard deviation (PSD) the differences between the measured field and the reference field are adjusted for the value of MD. These adjusted differences are then squared and again averaged across the field with each value weighted by its expected 'normal' variation. PSD attempts to estimate the non-uniform part of any deviation, as locations differing from the reference field by more than the value of MD will be empha-

sised by taking the square of adjusted differences. PSD is always positive and increases when localised field defects develop and progress. In Fig. 5.5 PSD is 3.16 dB and less than 10% of 'normal' fields from a patient of this age would exhibit a PSD value of at least this size.

Short-term fluctuation

SF is the standard deviation at 10 predetermined locations where the threshold is determined twice. It is an estimate of the repeatability of the patient's responses. In Fig. 5.5, the within test variability is 1.44 dB, which indicates a patient with reliable responses.

Corrected pattern standard deviation

Corrected pattern standard deviation (CPSD) estimates that part of PSD which is not attributed to SF. CPSD aims to differentiate between real deviations and those due to within test variability.

$$CPSD^2 = PSD^2 - k \times SF^2$$

Where k is a constant specified within STATPAC.

Other options available

Glaucoma Hemifield Test

Glaucoma Hemifield Test (GHT) is an optional analysis that tests for a difference in sensitivity between the superior and inferior hemifields. It compares the pattern deviation values in five sectors in the superior field with the mirror image in the inferior field. These sectors have been chosen to mimic the distribution of the nerve fibre bundles. However, even if the GHT test is outside 'normal' limits it does not necessarily mean that the field is in fact glaucomatous (see Chapter 7).

Overview and change analysis

STATPAC's overview printout can show the results of up to 16 field tests in chronological order. Four formats are plotted: gray scale, numeric, total deviation and pattern deviation. Like the overview, the change analysis shows the STATPAC analysis of up to 16 field tests. For

Table 5.2   **Advantages and disadvantages of automated perimetry**

Advantages	Disadvantages
Accurate: in the sense that testing conditions are reproducible	Learning
Stimulus parameters are standardised and can be varied	Fatigue
Examination strategy is known and reproducible	Testing can be time consuming, especially with the older full-threshold algorithms which take even longer to complete if there is a field defect
No observer bias affecting patient responses	Expensive
Computer software allows data storage and analysis	Ideally need separate room for instrumentation
Can be adapted to each individual patient	If performed by technical staff, they require appropriate training and re-training
Examination can be delegated to non-qualified staff	

example, STATPAC can perform a linear regression analysis on the mean deviation if between 5 and 16 central threshold field tests are available. It tests whether there is a statistically significant linear trend in mean deviation over time. One of two messages is displayed, 'MD slope not significant' or 'MD slope significant' (see Chapter 7).

5.8 SUMMARY

Modern automated perimeters can generate a great deal of information for each visual field test, and the various plots and indices described in this chapter are attempts to simplify the interpretation of these results. It is likely that in co-management schemes guidelines would be devised which are instrument specific.[28,29] Systematically examining the various reliability and global indices and the accompanying field plots assists in deciding whether pathological field loss is present or progressing, while also taking account of the effects of learning, fatigue and between and within test variability (Table 5.2). In uncertain cases it is always advisable to repeat the visual field test on another occasion.

The examples (Figs 5.6–5.10) that follow are from glaucomatous patients, and the reliability indices are remarkably good in all cases because

Fig. 5.6   The testing of this patient's right eye took 10 minutes and 11 seconds using the central 24-2 full threshold programme. The fixation was steady, as there are no reported fixation losses. Mean deviation (MD) shows that the field is depressed by 11.44 dB on average, which is most unlikely to occur in a 'normal' field (p < 0.5% for MD). This depression of the field is reflected in the low threshold values in the numerical plot of retinal sensitivity, and shown more clearly in the numerical and gray symbol total deviation plots. The probability of such low threshold values occurring in a 'normal' individual is less than 0.5% for the majority of the locations tested. In contrast, the pattern deviation plots show that only a few locations are depressed by more than the average and pattern standard deviation (PSD) = 2.22 dB, indicating subtle localised loss. There are five locations in the lower temporal quadrant forming a localised defect (in addition to the generalised loss of sensitivity) and threshold levels at least this extreme would be expected in less than 1% of 'normal' fields at three locations, less than 2% at one location, and less than 5% at the location closest to fixation. In summary, there is considerable generalised loss of sensitivity, together with localised loss limited to one quadrant. The reliability of the patient responses is good (short-term fluctuation (SF) = 1.02 dB). CPSD is similar to PSD because only a small proportion of PSD can be attributed to the SF. This visual field was from a patient with quite dense cataract and primary open angle glaucoma.

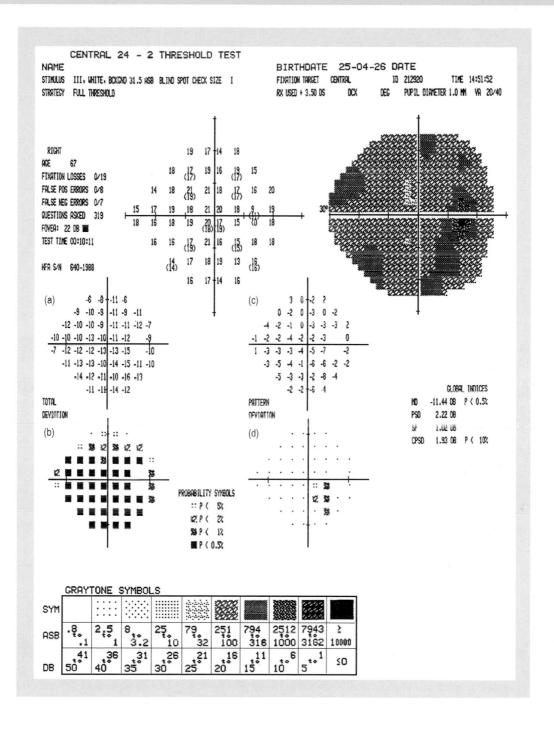

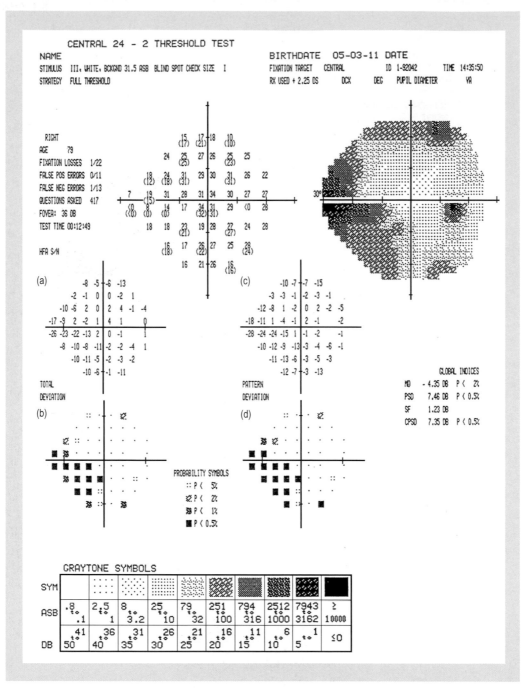

Fig. 5.7 Full threshold HFA 24-2 programme. In this patient the total and pattern deviation plots look similar, which indicates that most of the reduction in sensitivity is localised and not due to an overall depression of the field. The field is asymmetric, affecting the lower nasal quadrant predominantly with few locations affected above the midline. The mean deviation (MD) is not as depressed in this patient as in the previous example but the pattern standard deviation (PSD) is much higher. This glaucomatous field is showing primarily localised loss in the lower hemifield. The field is on average depressed by 4.35 dB (but the contribution to the calculation of MD is mainly due to those depressed locations in the lower field) and there is a deep localised depression. On average, locations deviate from the age matched normal values (the age reference) by 7.58 dB after allowing for any overall depression or suprasensitivity of the field. The patient's responses are reliable as indicated by short-term fluctuation (SF) of 1.23 dB, and therefore CPSD and PSD are numerically very similar. Values for CPSD and PSD as extreme as this would be expected to occur in less than 0.5% of 'normal' individuals.

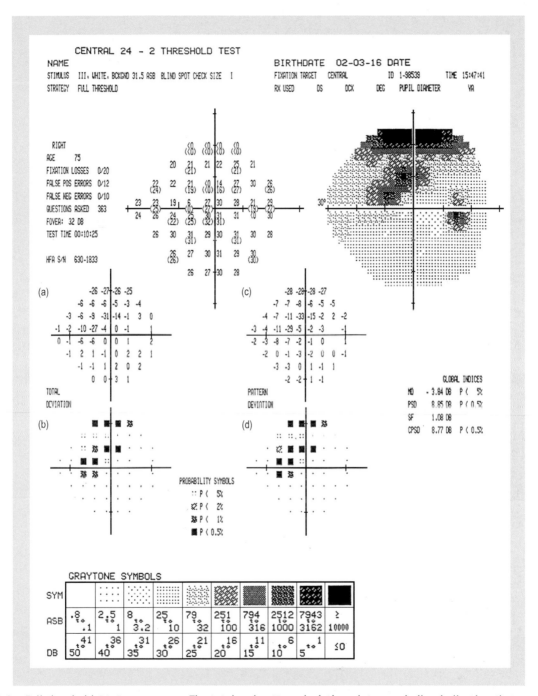

Fig. 5.8 Full threshold 24-2 programme. The total and pattern deviation plots are similar, indicating that once we allow for the overall depression in the field of 3.84 dB, there are locations remaining which are depressed by considerably more than this, as shown by the PSD of 8.85 dB. This indicates that, on average, locations deviate from the age matched normal values (the age reference) by 8.85 dB after allowing for any overall depression or suprasensitivity of the field. These values are unlikely to be observed in a 'normal' field. The upper hemifield is predominantly affected with a typical arcuate defect. Once again this patient's responses are reliable with short-term fluctuation (SF) = 1.08 dB.

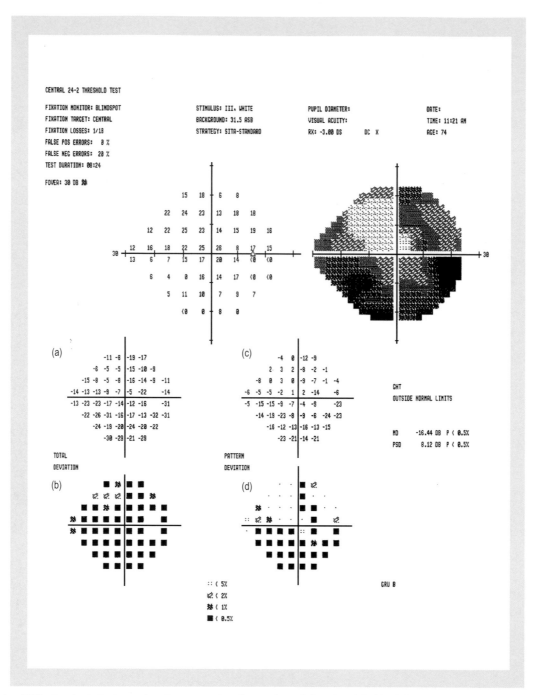

Fig. 5.9 SITA standard strategy showing extensive depression of the visual field with a mean deviation (MD) of −16.44 dB. Both the total and pattern deviation plots show involvement of both hemifields, although there is more localised loss in the lower hemifield (as shown in the pattern deviation plot) and the Glaucoma Hemifield Test (GHT, see Chapter 7 for more details on this test) is stated as being 'outside normal limits'. The pattern standard deviation (PSD) is high and a value at least as extreme as 8.12 dB is most unlikely to occur in a 'normal' population (<0.5% of 'normal' individuals).

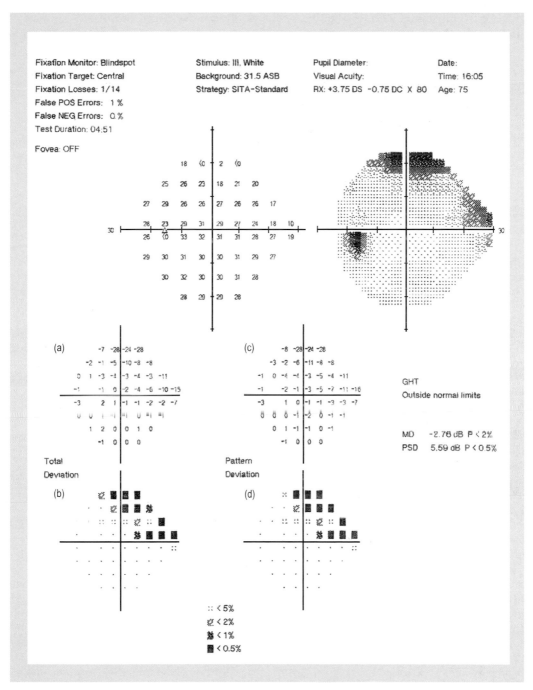

Fig. 5.10 SITA standard central 24-2 programme showing an arcuate defect in the superior field. There may be the onset of a field defect involving the inferior hemifield with one location identified with a probability of <5% in the total and pattern deviation plots. The Glaucoma Hemifield Test (GHT) is outside 'normal' limits and although the mean deviation (MD) value is moderately depressed (−2.76 dB) the value for PSD is 5.59 dB, a value that would be expected to occur in less than 0.5% of 'normal' individuals, indicating the predominately localised nature of this glaucomatous field defect.

these fields are from patients who were very experienced in automated perimetry.

5.9 OTHER VARIANTS OF AUTOMATED PERIMETRY

The following are alternative perimetric testing methods that have been investigated for use in glaucoma, and they are discussed in Chapter 6.

- Short-wavelength automated perimetry (SWAP) —also known as blue-on-yellow perimetry, or short wavelength sensitive perimetry
- Frequency doubling perimetry
- High pass resolution perimetry
- Flicker perimetry
- Motion perimetry
- Pattern discrimination perimetry.

Many of the above are still under investigation and are not used routinely in clinical practice.

References

1. Greve EL. Single and multiple stimulus static perimetry in glaucoma; the two phases of the visual field examination. Doc Ophthalmol 1973; 36:1–355.
2. Heijl A, Krakau CET. An automatic perimeter, design and pilot study. Acta Ophthalmol 1975; 53:293–310.
3. Wood JM, Wild JM, Hussey M, et al. Serial examination of the 'normal' visual field using Octopus projection perimetry: evidence of a learning effect. Acta Ophthalmol 1987; 65:326–333.
4. Heijl A, Lindgren G, Olsson J. The effect of perimetric experience in 'normal' subjects. Arch Ophthalmol 1989; 107:81–86.
5. Wild JM, Dengler-Harles M, Searle AET, et al. The influence of the learning effect on automated perimetry in patients with suspected glaucoma. Acta Ophthalmol 1989; 67:537–545.
6. Guttridge NM, Allen PM, Rudnicka AR, et al. Influence of learning on the peripheral field as assessed by automated perimetry. In: Mills RP, Heijl A, eds. Perimetry Update 1990/1991. Amstelveen: Kugler and Ghedini; 1991:567–575.
7. Heijl, A. Time changes of contrast thresholds during automated perimetry. Acta Ophthalmol 1977; 55:696–708.
8. Holmin C, Krakau CET. Variability of glaucomatous visual field defects in computerised perimetry. Graefes Arch Clin Exp Ophthalmol 1979; 210:235–250.
9. Heijl A, Drance SM. Changes in differential light threshold in patients with glaucoma during prolonged perimetry. Br J Ophthalmol 1983; 67:512–516.
10. Johnson CA, Adams CW, Lewis RA. Fatigue effects in automated perimetry. Appl Opt 1988; 27:1030–1037.
11. Langerhorst C, van den Berg TJTP, Veldman E, et al. Population study of global and local fatigue with prolonged threshold testing in automated perimetry. Doc Ophthalmol Proc Ser 1987; 49:657–662.
12. Rudnicka AR, Crabb DP, Edgar DF, et al. Pointwise analysis of serial visual fields in 'normal' subjects. In: Heijl A, Mills RP, eds. Perimetry Update 1992/1993. Amsterdam: Kugler Publications; 1993:41–48.
13. Jaffe GJ, Alvarado JA, Juster RP. Age related changes of the 'normal' visual field. Arch Ophthalmol 1986; 104:1021–1025.
14. Nelson-Quigg JM, Twelker JD, Johnson CA. Response properties of 'normal' observers and patients during automated perimetry. Arch Ophthalmol 1989; 107:1612–1615.
15. Flammer J, Drance SM, Zulauf M. Differential light threshold. Short- and long-term fluctuations in patients with glaucoma, 'normal' controls and patients with suspected glaucoma. Arch Ophthalmol 1984; 102:704–706.
16. Flammer J, Drance SM, Fankhauser F, et al. Differential light threshold in automatic threshold perimetry: factors influencing the short-term fluctuation. Arch Ophthalmol 1984; 102:876–879.
17. Henson DB. Visual Fields. Oxford: Butterworth Heinemann; 2000.
18. Henson DB, Anderson RS. Threshold-related suprathreshold visual field testing: which is the best technique of establishing the threshold? In: Mills RP, Heijl A, eds. Perimetry Update 1990/1991.

Amstelveen: Kugler and Ghedini; 1991:367–372.

19. Henson DB, Artes P. New developments in supra-threshold perimetry. Ophthalmic and Physiol Opt 2002; 22:463–468.

20. Bengtsson B, Olsson J, Rootzen H. A new generation of algorithms for computerized perimetry, SITA. Acta Ophthalmol 1997; 75:368–375.

21. Wild J. SITA—a new outlook for visual field examination in primary shared care. Optician 1997; March 14: 213.

22. Bengtsson B, Heijl A. Evaluation of a new threshold visual field threshold strategy, SITA, in 'subjects'. Acta Ophthalmol 1998; 76:165–169.

23. Bengtsson B, Heijl A. Evaluation of a new perimetric threshold strategy, SITA, in patients with manifest and suspect glaucoma. Acta Ophthalmol 1998; 76:268–272.

24. Bengtsson B, Heijl A. SITA FAST, a new rapid perimetric threshold test. Description of methods and evaluation in patients with manifest and suspect glaucoma. Acta Ophthalmol 1998; 76:431–437.

25. Bengtsson B, Heijl A. Comparing significance and magnitude of glaucomatous visual field defects using the SITA and Full threshold strategies. Acta Ophthalmol Scand 1999; 77:143–146.

26. Wild J, Pacey IE, Hancock SA. Between-algorithm, between-individual differences in 'normal' perimetric sensitivity: full threshold, FASTPAC, and SITA. Invest Ophthalmol Vis Sci 1999; 40:1152–1161.

27. Sekhar GC, Naduvilath TJ, Lakkai M, et al. Sensitivity of Swedish interactive threshold algorithm compared with standard full threshold algorithm in Humphrey visual field. Ophthalmology 2000; 107:1303–1308.

28. Henson DB, Darling MN. Detecting progressive visual field loss. Ophthalmic Physiol Opt 1995; 15:387–390.

29. Henson DB, Spry PG, Spencer IC, et al. Variability in glaucomatous visual fields: implications for shared care schemes. Ophthalmic Physiol Opt 1998; 18:120–125.

Chapter 6

Visual function in glaucoma

David Thomson

6.1 INTRODUCTION

The function of the retina is to sample the retinal image and convert this information into a form that may be conveyed to the visual areas of the brain. This process is mediated by a rich network of retinal neurones that ultimately outputs a complex transformation of the retinal image to approximately one million nerve fibres that funnel through the optic nerve head. The term 'glaucoma' is used to describe a group of pathological conditions that cause progressive damage to these nerve fibres. It is not surprising that damage to this complex conduit of visual information can have subtle and variable effects on visual function.

The effects of glaucoma on differential light sensitivity across the visual field are well documented and still form the basis of the clinical diagnosis.[1] In the early stages of the disease, the areas of reduced sensitivity (scotomas) are small and relative but, as the disease progresses, the scotomas deepen, expand and coalesce until, in extreme cases, there is a complete loss of visual function over the entire visual field.

The subtle loss in sensitivity during the early stages of glaucoma usually goes unnoticed and in the absence of any other symptoms, patients are normally unaware of their condition until the field defects are quite advanced, by which stage significant and irreversible damage has occurred. For this reason, a great deal of research has gone into the early detection of the disease. Until relatively recently, much of this research focused on the detection of ever-more subtle changes in sensitivity across the visual field. This work led to the development of a variety of sophisticated instruments and psychophysical algorithms, which have greatly improved the sensitivity and specificity of visual field screening.

However, over the past 20 years there has been a growing body of evidence to suggest that significant nerve fibre damage can occur before changes are detected by even the most sensitive visual field tests.[2] It has also become apparent that some aspects of visual function may be reduced before the appearance of visual field defects and that visual function outside scotomas (including central vision) can show specific functional deficits when probed with appropriate stimuli.[3]

These findings have stimulated the drive to develop alternative screening tests so that the disease process can be detected and treated at an earlier stage. The rationale behind many of the newer tests has been the finding by Quigley et al[4] that larger nerve fibres are more susceptible to damage in the early stages of glaucoma. Such fibres are functionally, as well as anatomically, distinct from the smaller fibres; the two types of fibre being responsible for conveying information about different spatio-temporal components of the retinal image. The working hypothesis has been that selective damage to the large fibres may lead to a specific visual deficit while other aspects of visual function remain unaffected.

6.2 THE PARVO AND MAGNO PATHWAYS

To understand the nature of these changes, it is necessary to consider the functional organisation of the retina and the visual pathway.

The primate retina contains at least 20 different types of ganglion cell.[5] *In vitro* preparations of the primate retina show three types of ganglion cell projecting to the lateral geniculate nucleus (LGN): the parasol, midget and small bi-stratified cells. The morphology, physiology and projections of these cells have been studied extensively.[6,7] The axon diameter is related to cell size, which in turn increases with eccentricity for all types of ganglion cell. At any given eccentricity the parasol cells tend

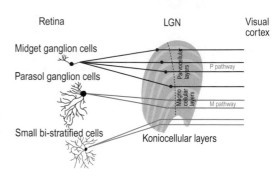

Fig. 6.1 Schematic representation of the Parvo and Magno pathways.

to be larger than the midget cells. The parasol cells also tend to have larger dendritic fields than the midget cells.

The majority of parasol cells project to the magnocellular layers (1 and 2) of the LGN whereas most midget cells project to the parvocellular layers (3–6).[8] There is some evidence that the small bi-stratified cells project to the koniocellular layers of the LGN[9] (Fig. 6.1). The segregation of the fibres continues from the LGN to the primary visual cortex and to some extent beyond this in the dorsal and ventral streams. This concept of two anatomically and functionally distinct pathways conveying information from the retina to the brain is now well established.[10] The two pathways tend to be referred to as the **P** and **M** systems according to whether they project via the **P**arvocellular or the **M**agnocellular layers of the LGN.

There are considerable differences between the physiological properties of the two pathways.[11–13] Electrophysiological studies in primates have shown that the P system conveys information about colour and is characterised by good spatial resolution (acuity) but poor temporal resolution (i.e. it is unable to respond to rapid changes). In contrast, the M system has good temporal sensitivity and contrast sensitivity, but is achromatic and has poor spatial resolution. The functional specialisation of the two pathways is supported by behavioural studies of monkeys with ablated sections of the LGN. Recent research suggests that blue-yellow colour vision is mediated by the small bi-stratified ganglion cells and red-green colour vision by the P ganglion cells.[9]

The M and P systems derive their different spatio-temporal properties by virtue of differences in their preganglionic connectivity and, to some extent, differences between the characteristics of the ganglion cells subserving the two systems. Approximately 90% of ganglion cells project to the parvocellular layers of the LGN. Although P ganglion cells are found throughout the retina, their density decreases with eccentricity. The receptive field size of both P and M ganglion cells varies with eccentricity but in general the M cell receptive fields are larger than those of the P cells. The axons from the M ganglion cells are generally larger than those of the P cells and therefore selective damage of the large fibres may produce a deficit in M function before there is any change in the properties of the P system.

6.3 THE NATURE OF GLAUCOMATOUS DAMAGE

There is strong clinical and histological evidence that nerve fibres at the superior and inferior poles of the optic nerve head tend to be more susceptible to glaucomatous damage.[4,14–16] This results in the characteristic arcuate field defects (see section 5.5) in 'early' glaucoma.

In addition, a number of studies have found that, at a given location within the optic nerve head, the large nerve fibres are lost at a faster rate than the smaller nerve fibres. For example, Quigley et al[4] induced chronic glaucoma in 10 monkeys and compared the optic nerves of the glaucomatous eyes and the normal fellow eyes. They reported that there was a preferential loss of large diameter axons regardless of the location within the optic nerve. Similar results have been found when comparing post-mortem human eyes with glaucoma and age-matched post-enucleated normal eyes.

It is not clear why large fibres appear to be particularly susceptible in glaucoma. It has been suggested that it is due to the fact that they are found mainly in the superior and inferior poles of the optic nerve head, areas that are known to be weaker and susceptible to damage in glaucoma. An alternative suggestion is that in eyes with elevated intraocular pressure (IOP), the absorption of nutrients from the axon membrane is decreased due to reduced tissue perfusion.[17,18] This would tend to affect the large fibres more because of their larger surface-to-volume ratio.

The evidence for preferential large fibre loss is persuasive but not conclusive.[19] It is also important to note that axon diameter increases with retinal eccentricity for both P and M cells and the axons of some peripheral P cells may in fact be larger than some more central M cells. It is also wrong to assume the P cells are immune to early damage.

However, it is reasonable to conclude that neural loss in glaucoma is partially selective for the M pathway and therefore some deficits in the aspects of visual function mediated by this pathway may be expected in the early stages of glaucoma.

6.4 VISUAL FUNCTION IN GLAUCOMA

The most widely used test for assessing visual function in glaucoma is static perimetry. The task for the patient is to detect small white stimuli superimposed on a uniform white background at discrete points within the visual field. Ideally, the differential luminance threshold at each point is determined giving a map of relative sensitivity across the visual field which can then be searched for patterns of reduced sensitivity that are considered typical of glaucoma. Modern instruments employ a variety of algorithms in a bid to minimise the number of presentations required to determine a reliable estimate of the threshold at each point.

The clinical diagnosis of glaucoma is currently based on the presence of field loss, assessment of the optic disc and consideration of risk factors such as elevated IOP, family history, race, etc. However, there is now good evidence that between 20% and 40% of ganglion cells may be lost before field defects are detected by conventional visual field analysis.[2,16] This is presumably partly attributable to the fact that the small white stimuli used in perimetry are likely to stimulate both P and M cells and are unlikely to detect early deficits in the M system.

In view of this, numerous studies have sought to develop stimuli and tests that will detect glaucomatous damage at an earlier stage.[3] Some have specifically targeted the P system, some have sought to compare P and M function, but in view of the evidence that M pathway deficits may occur first, most have attempted to probe the properties of the M system.

6.4.1 VISUAL FUNCTION IN THE FOVEAL AND PARA-FOVEAL REGIONS

It is generally considered that vision in the central five degrees is unaffected in glaucoma until the final stages of the disease when the field defects approach fixation. However, there is growing evidence that certain aspects of visual function in this part of the visual field may be affected at an earlier stage. Changes in visual function in the central visual field are of particular interest due to the importance of this area in determining the overall quality of functional vision.

6.4.2 SPATIAL CONTRAST SENSITIVITY

Since the pioneering work of Campbell[20,21] and others in the 1960s, contrast sensitivity (CS) testing has emerged as a valuable technique in the evaluation of the spatial properties of vision.

The minimum contrast for an observer to detect a pattern is the measure of contrast threshold – CS is the reciprocal of contrast threshold. CS can be measured for a target of any shape or size; however the use of sinusoidal gratings is preferable if precise information is sought for specific sizes (spatial frequencies). Sinusoidal gratings are usually presented on television-type displays under computer control. CS is determined by varying the contrast of the grating until the subject reports that the grating is just visible/not visible. This is usually repeated at a number of spatial frequencies and the results plotted in the form of a contrast sensitivity function (CSF) as shown in Fig. 6.2.

Visual acuity can be estimated from the high spatial frequency cut-off of the CSF. A variety of chart-based systems for measuring CS have been developed including the Pelli-Robson chart, low contrast acuity charts and the Cambridge Grating Test. While these tests do not allow a complete CSF to be constructed, they do provide a second point on the function which may be valuable in the evaluation of certain types of visual loss.

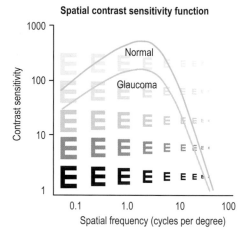

Fig. 6.2   The spatial contrast sensitivity function.

Many studies have found that spatial contrast sensitivity is reduced in patients with glaucoma.[22-31] The nature of the CS loss seems to be variable but most studies report the greatest reduction at intermediate spatial frequencies (Fig. 6.2). The prevalence of significant CS loss reported in the literature varies between 50% and 93% for patients with glaucoma[28,29] and between 20% and 70% for patients with ocular hypertension.[31]

The loss of spatial CS at intermediate spatial frequencies suggests that some glaucoma patients may experience a reduction in the quality of their central vision even in the absence of central scotomas. It also explains why high contrast visual acuity is usually normal in glaucoma and suggests that Pelli-Robson CS or low contrast visual acuity may be useful additional tests to perform in clinical practice. Unfortunately, the range of CS in glaucoma is wide and there is a great deal of overlap between glaucomatous and normal populations. CS testing is therefore of limited value for screening but does provide a better indication of patients' visual status than high contrast visual acuity.

Improved specificity can be obtained if the grating is moved or temporally-modulated (flickered). Atkin et al[23] compared several spatial and temporal frequencies of modulation and concluded that low spatial frequency patterns modulated in time at about 8 Hz provide the best statistical discrimination between normal subjects and glaucoma patients. It is interesting to note that these test conditions are likely to favour the M system.

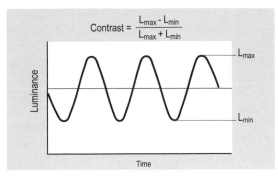

Fig. 6.3 The luminance of a uniform field is modulated sinusoidally in time. The minimum modulation (contrast) required to perceive flicker is measured at various frequencies to construct a temporal contrast sensitivity function.

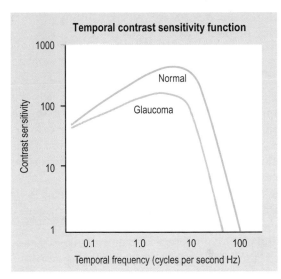

Fig. 6.4 Temporal contrast sensitivity is often reduced in glaucoma, particularly at higher frequencies.

6.4.3 TEMPORAL CONTRAST SENSITIVITY

Temporal CS is determined by presenting a spatially uniform field, which is modulated (flickered) sinusoidally in time. The degree of modulation (temporal contrast) is varied until the patient reports that flicker is just perceptible (Fig. 6.3). This is usually repeated for a range of flicker frequencies and the results plotted in a similar form to the spatial contrast sensitivity function (except the abscissa now refers to temporal frequency in Hz; Fig. 6.4). Maximum sensitivity (minimum modulation required to detect flicker) usually occurs for frequencies in the range of 5–15 Hz. In glaucoma, sensitivity for middle and higher frequencies is often impaired.[32–34] Again it is interesting to note that the perception of flicker at these frequencies is likely to be mediated by the M pathway.

Unlike tasks of spatial discrimination, temporal sensitivity is relatively immune to degradation of the retinal image by refractive error or media opacities. However, other conditions such as maculopathy can affect temporal sensitivity and for this reason the test may be of more value for screening when applied in the peripheral field (see later).

6.4.4 COLOUR VISION

Losses in colour sensitivity, particularly discriminations mediated by the short-wavelength-sensitive (blue) cones, are often noted in patients with glaucoma and these losses can occur before the onset of visual field defects in ocular hypertensive subjects.[35–45] Kelly et al[42] found that 26% of the glaucoma patients they tested had a significant reduction in red-green discrimination and 42% were significantly deficient at yellow-blue colour discrimination. Unfortunately, such colour vision defects are not easily detected by conventional colour vision tests.

The reduction in blue cone sensitivity seems to be particularly apparent in the peripheral visual field and may precede the development of scotomas (demonstrable by conventional white on white perimetry). This is discussed in a later section.

6.4.5 VISUAL FUNCTION IN THE MORE PERIPHERAL VISUAL FIELD

White-on-white perimetry

The principal change in visual function in glaucoma is a loss of sensitivity in the visual field. This can be demonstrated by measuring differential light sensitivity at discrete points in the visual field. Field loss tends to follow a characteristic pattern which has been described in detail in Chapter 5 and by Drance.[46] However, as described earlier, it is evident that significant neural damage can occur before field defects are apparent using white-on-white perimetry.

Blue-on-yellow perimetry

Visual field testing using coloured (especially blue) stimuli has been reported to be superior to using conventional white targets.[47-51] The blue cones can be isolated by using a yellow background (which reduces the sensitivity of the medium (green) and long-wavelength-sensitive (red) cones), and selecting a blue target of an appropriate wavelength (less than 475 nm). The yellow background also serves to minimise the contribution from the rods. A number of commercial instruments may be modified for blue-on-yellow testing (also known as short wavelength automated perimetry or SWAP).

Glaucomatous visual field defects identified by blue-on-yellow perimetry often precede defects found by white-on-white perimetry. Defects identified by the two methods tend to be in the same area of the visual field although blue-on-yellow defects are often larger and show a faster rate of progression (Fig. 6.5). Therefore, blue-on-yellow perimetry shows considerable promise for the early detection of glaucoma. However, the intra-test and inter-patient variability tends to be rather greater than for conventional perimetry and blue-on-yellow thresholds have been shown to increase with age (particularly after 50 years). This is probably attributable to the 'yellowing' of the crystalline lens.

It is not clear if the susceptibility of the blue system to damage in early glaucoma is due to the relative scarcity of blue cones or rather to some form of selective preganglionic damage. It is also possible that the axons from the small bi-stratified ganglion cells (which are thought to mediate blue-yellow vision) may be particularly susceptible to damage in glaucoma.

Flicker perimetry

Flicker sensitivity can be assessed in the peripheral field by measuring temporal contrast sensitivity at various flicker rates (as described above). Alternatively, the highest detectable flicker rate (flicker fusion frequency, FFF) can be measured at a number of discrete positions in the visual field.

Flicker perimetry may be carried out using a computer monitor or using a modified perimeter that permits the stimuli to be flashed at different frequencies. Flicker thresholds are abnormal in most patients with chronic open-angle glaucoma.[32,52-55] The loss in flicker sensitivity occurs across the range of temporal frequencies but tends to be greater at high frequencies. Several authors have reported that flicker perimetry is reduced in a high proportion of patients with ocular hypertension and may have some value in predicting which patients are likely to develop glaucoma.[56,57]

Flicker thresholds are relatively immune to image blurring and degradation but do increase with age.[58,59] Flicker perimetry shows some promise as a screening test but further studies are required to establish the optimum stimulus parameters.

Frequency-doubling perimetry

The frequency-doubling illusion occurs when a low spatial frequency grating is counter-phase modulated at a high temporal frequency (i.e. the contrast of the bars is rapidly reversed). This phenomenon was first described by Kelly[60] and subsequently evaluated by many other investigators. The perception of this stimulus is likely to be mediated principally by mechanisms in the M-cell pathway, possibly a subset of ganglion cells known as M_y cells.

Johnson and Samuels[61,62] argued that such a stimulus is ideally suited to probe M cell function in glaucoma and developed a system known as frequency-doubling technology (FDT) (Fig. 6.6). The instrument presents a $10 \times 10°$ low-spatial frequency grating (0.25 cycles/deg) consisting of black and white bars undergoing a rapid counter-phase modulation (25 Hz). The gratings are presented at 16 locations within the visual field and the patient is simply required to respond if they can detect the grating against the uniform gray background. The contrast threshold for the detection of the flickering grating is compared with age-matched norms.

A screening test can be performed in less than 2 minutes per eye and thresholds can be determined in approximately 5 minutes. Glaucoma patients fail to detect the stimuli in regions that grossly match the part of the visual field found to be defective by

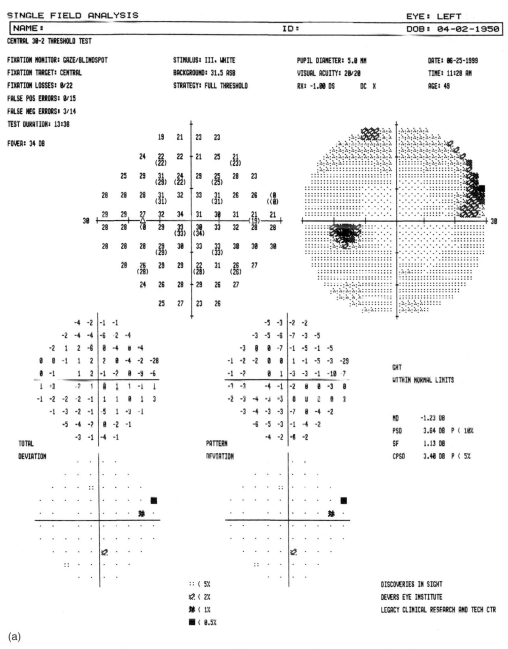

Fig. 6.5a Field plots for a patient using white-on-white perimetry. (Source: Humphrey instruments; www.humphrey.com)

conventional perimetry. The instrument is fast and appears to have good sensitivity and specificity for glaucoma screening. It also offers the possibility of being able to detect changes in visual function before conventional perimetry although its efficacy in this respect has not been fully established.[63–69]

Motion perimetry

The perception of certain types of motion is thought to be mediated by the M pathway and a number of studies have tested the hypothesis that motion perception may be affected in the early

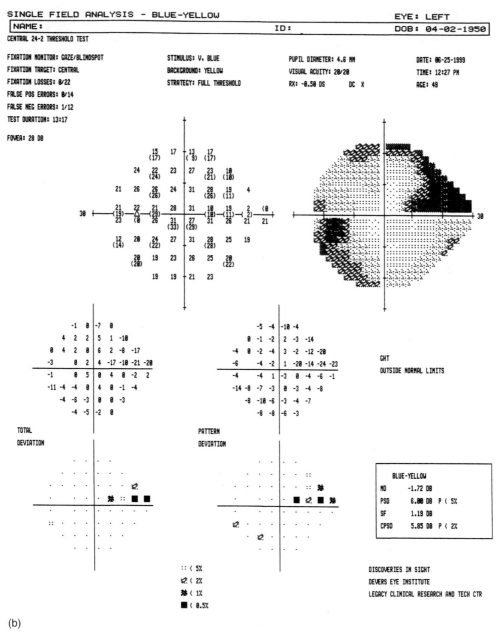

(b)

Fig, 6.5b Field plots for the same patient using blue-on-yellow perimetry. Scotomas are often apparent using blue-on-yellow perimetry before they are detected by conventional perimetry. (Source: Humphrey instruments; www.humphrey.com)

stages of glaucoma.[70] A wide range of stimuli and methodologies have been used to assess motion perception. The tests can be broadly divided into global (full field) and local (at specific locations in the visual field). Various aspects of motion processing have been assessed including motion detection, direction discrimination, motion localisation and thresholds for the detection of coherent motion among an array of randomly moving dots.[71–76]

An alternative approach is to measure the minimum displacement (displacement threshold) required to perceive the oscillatory motion of a bar or spot target.[73,77,78] In general, motion perimetry reveals a decrease in motion sensitivity in regions of the visual field that grossly match the areas of field loss found by conventional perimetry. Some aspects of motion processing in the peripheral visual field have also been shown to be affected during the early stages of glaucoma prior to detectable field loss.

Determining the potential value of motion perimetry as a screening test for glaucoma is difficult because of the wide range of stimulus config-

urations used and the corresponding variation in the tests' sensitivity and specificity. However, some studies have now demonstrated tests with excellent sensitivity and specificity and motion perimetry can be considered as a promising diagnostic tool. Longitudinal studies are now required to determine if eyes demonstrating decreased motion thresholds will eventually develop field defects and what is currently defined as glaucoma.

Other forms of perimetry

Many other stimuli have been proposed for detecting visual field deficits in glaucoma. Many have been shown to offer little over conventional perimetry but two are worthy of further consideration.

High-pass resolution perimetry

High-pass resolution perimetry is a test of peripheral spatial resolution and therefore targets the P type retinal ganglion cells. It is thought to provide an indirect measure of the number of functioning ganglion cells and is therefore of value for detecting a relative loss of ganglion cells in glaucoma.[79]

The stimulus for high-pass resolution perimetry is a light annulus with dark borders presented on a gray background (Fig. 6.7). The space-averaged

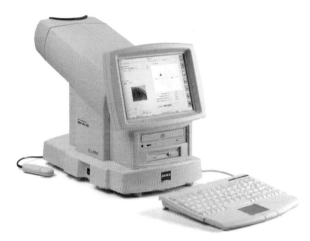

Fig. 6.6   The Humphrey FDT visual field instrument. (Source: Humphrey instruments; www.humphrey.com)

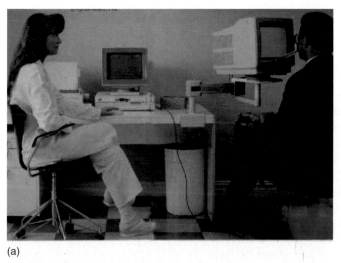
(a)

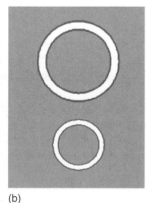
(b)

Fig. 6.7ab   In high-pass resolution perimetry, an annulus is presented in different parts of the visual field and the minimum diameter for detection is measured. (Source of Fig.6.7a: Visumetrics; www.visumetrics.com)

luminance of the ring is matched to the background so that the detection and resolution thresholds are very similar – targets are either seen and resolved or invisible.

The stimulus is presented at various locations within the visual field and the size of the annulus is varied to determine the resolution threshold. The test can be performed with good reliability in 6–8 minutes for 50 locations within the visual field.

In general, high-pass resolution thresholds are increased in glaucoma and there is good concordance with conventional perimetry with respect to the location and depth of scotomas. Some studies have found disturbances in high-pass resolution fields before the appearance of field defects while others have not.[80–86]

High-pass resolution perimetry is reported to be a robust test with good test-retest repeatability. However, long-term studies are needed to demonstrate its value as a screening test for early glaucoma.

Pattern discrimination perimetry

Pattern discrimination perimetry was developed by Drum et al.[87] It is based on the assumption that the perception of fine patterns is formulated from the integrated response of all the ganglion cells whose receptive fields are sampling the pattern. Any loss of ganglion cells would result in a reduction in the ability to discriminate a pattern against its background.

The clinical implementation of this test involves presenting a regular chequerboard pattern of black and white squares against a background array of random black and white squares that are constantly changing. The normal visual system is remarkably good at discriminating the pattern from the background 'noise'. Threshold is measured by varying the stimulus coherence (where 100% represents a pure chequerboard and 0% is identical to the background). Theoretically, a loss in ganglion cell density will result in a reduction in pattern discrimination and an increase in coherence thresholds. The test is implemented on a computer screen and the size of the squares is increased with eccentricity to balance the effect of the corresponding decrease in ganglion cell density.

In general, pattern discrimination thresholds are increased in glaucoma and there is a reasonable correlation with conventional perimetry in terms of the location and depth of scotomas.[88–92] Pattern discrimination thresholds have also been reported to be raised in approximately half of ocular hypertensives but further longitudinal studies are required to determine the true value of this technique in detecting early neural loss in glaucoma.

6.4.6 OBJECTIVE TESTS OF VISUAL FUNCTION

The tests described thus far require the patient to make a series of subjective responses. This can be arduous, particularly for older patients, and results are often variable due to the effects of learning, fatigue, etc. This has led to renewed interest in electrophysiological tests in relation to the detection of glaucoma, in particular the electroretinogram.

An electroretinogram (ERG) is a recording of the transient change in the standing potential of the eye in response to visual stimulation. An ERG is recorded by placing the active electrode on or close to the cornea and a reference electrode on a relatively inactive site, usually the forehead (Fig. 6.8). The ERG is a complex response arising from potentials generated in a variety of retinal cells. The shape of the ERG depends on many factors, in particular the nature of the retinal stimulation and the state of retinal adaptation. Its clinical value arises from the fact that both the shape and

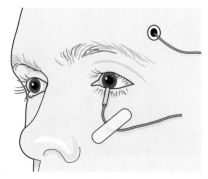

Fig. 6.8 Measuring an electroretinogram using a gold-leaf corneal electrode.

amplitude of the response are affected in a number of retinal diseases.

Historically, most investigators have used flashes of light to generate ERG responses. Although the shape of the flash ERG depends on many factors, three main components, known as the a, b and c waves, can usually be identified. These components are derived mainly from the photoreceptors, the bipolar cells and the retinal pigment epithelium, respectively, none of which are specifically affected in the early stages of glaucoma. Consequently, while there is some evidence that the amplitude of the flash ERG is affected in glaucoma, the effects are small and are not apparent until the later stages of the disease.

Riggs et al[93] were among the first to study the ERG to patterned stimuli. Some years later, a resurgence of interest in pattern stimulation was sparked by new evidence that pattern ERGs (PERGs) may reflect activity at a more proximal level in the retina than the flash ERG.[94,95] Maffei and colleagues demonstrated that the PERG gradually disappeared following section of the optic nerve, suggesting that the response was, at least in part, mediated by retinal ganglion cells, (ganglion cell activity does not contribute significantly to the flash ERG).[94,95] Since then, a wide variety of patterned stimuli have been used including gratings, bars and checks. Usually, the pattern is periodically reversed so that the black areas become white and vice versa, while the overall luminance remains constant. The morphology of the PERG is dependent on a number of factors, particularly the configuration of the patterned stimulus.

The first reports of PERG abnormalities in glaucoma date from the early 1980s. Since then numerous studies have shown that the PERG is grossly reduced in glaucoma patients.[96–105] Furthermore, there is growing evidence that changes in the PERG can occur before the appearance of field defects.

The PERG has been shown to have good sensitivity as a screening test. However, the specificity is poor because many other conditions common in the glaucomatous age group such as age-related maculopathy, cataracts, diabetes, etc. can have similar effects on the PERG. Furthermore, the test requires sophisticated equipment and a high degree of cooperation from the patient. While the measurement of PERGs may be useful for studying the disease process and the effects of treatment, with present techniques it is unsuitable for general screening.

6.5 SUMMARY

Glaucoma causes diffuse and localised damage to the retinal nerve fibres. Each nerve fibre carries a complex transformation of the information contained within a small area of the retinal image. The nature of the transformation depends on the eccentricity and the characteristics of the source ganglion cell. The human retina contains at least 20 different types of ganglion cell, each coding the spatial, temporal and chromatic characteristics of the retinal image in slightly different ways. It is not surprising, therefore, that damage to the nerve fibres can have complex and variable effects on visual function.

The effects of glaucoma on differential light sensitivity across the visual field are well documented. However, there is now good evidence that field defects are not the only, or necessarily the first, change in visual function. Psychophysical evidence suggests that changes in flicker and motion sensitivity, pattern discrimination and colour vision can occur before changes in sensitivity can be detected using conventional perimetry. This is supported by histological and electrophysiological evidence confirming that significant nerve fibre loss can occur without there being a measurable effect on visual fields.

While deficits in some of these aspects of visual function tend to map onto similar areas of the visual field identified by conventional perimetry, the areas are often larger. Furthermore, a reduction in various aspects of central visual function can be demonstrated in many glaucoma patients despite retaining good visual acuity.

Histological evidence that large nerve fibres are preferentially affected in early glaucoma is supported by psychophysical evidence that aspects of vision thought to be mediated by these fibres are also affected at an early stage; specifically sensitivity to low spatial frequencies, high temporal frequencies and motion stimuli. Unlike scotomas, which have relatively well-defined spatial dimensions,

M-pathway deficits tend to be more diffuse and therefore can be identified by testing fewer points in the visual field.

The possibility of detecting nerve fibre damage at an earlier stage than is possible with conventional perimetry has led to a proliferation of tests based on the isolation of M function, some of which show some potential as screening tests for glaucoma. While it seems likely that earlier detection and treatment will result in less nerve fibre damage and subsequent field loss, the case is not yet proven.

References

1. Drance SM. Glaucomatous field defects. In: Rich R, Shields M, Krupin T, eds. The Glaucomas. St Louis: CV Mosby; 1989.
2. Quigley HA, Dunkelberger GR, Green WR. Retinal ganglion cell atrophy correlated with automated perimetry in human eyes with glaucoma. Am J Ophthalmol 1989; 107:453–464.
3. Stewart WC, Chauhan BC. Newer visual function tests in the evaluation of glaucoma. Surv Ophthalmol 1995; 40:119–135.
4. Quigley HA, Dunkelberger GR, Green WR. Chronic human glaucoma causing selectively greater loss of large optic nerve fibers. Ophthalmology 1988; 95:357–363.
5. Kolb H, Linberg KA, Fisher SK. Neurons of the human retina: a Golgi study. J Comp Neurol 1992; 318:147–187.
6. Rodieck RW, Watanabe M. Survey of the morphology of macaque retinal ganglion cells that project to the pretectum, superior colliculus, and parvicellular laminae of the lateral geniculate nucleus. J Comp Neurol 1993; 338:289–303.
7. Watanabe M, Rodieck RW. Parasol and midget ganglion cells of the primate retina. J Comp Neurol 1989; 289:434–454.
8. Perry VH, Oehler R, Cowey A. Retinal ganglion cells that project to the dorsal lateral geniculate nucleus in the macaque monkey. Neuroscience 1984; 12:1101–1123.
9. Dacey DM, Lee BB. The 'blue-on' opponent pathway in primate retina originates from a distinct bistratified ganglion cell type. Nature 1994; 367:731–735.
10. Lennie P. Parallel visual pathways: a review. Vision Res 1980; 20:561–594.
11. Croner LJ, Kaplan E. Receptive fields of P and M ganglion cells across the primate retina. Vision Res 1995; 35:7–24.
12. Benardete EA, Kaplan E, Knight BW. Contrast gain control in the primate retina: P cells are not X-like, some M cells are. Vis Neurosci 1992; 8:483–486.
13. Kaplan E, Shapley RM. The primate retina contains two types of ganglion cells, with high and low contrast sensitivity. Proc Natl Acad Sci USA 1986; 83:2755–2757.
14. Quigley HA. Early detection of glaucomatous damage. II. Changes in the appearance of the optic disk. Surv Ophthalmol 1985; 30:111–117, 126.
15. Quigley HA, Addicks EM, Green WR, et al. Optic nerve damage in human glaucoma. II. The site of injury and susceptibility to damage. Arch Ophthalmol 1981; 99:635–649.
16. Quigley HA, Addicks EM, Green WR. Optic nerve damage in human glaucoma. III. Quantitative correlation of nerve fiber loss and visual field defect in glaucoma, ischemic neuropathy, papilledema, and toxic neuropathy. Arch Ophthalmol 1982; 100:135–146.
17. Radius RL. Anatomy of the optic nerve head and glaucomatous optic neuropathy. Surv Ophthalmol 1987; 32:35–44.
18. Radius RL. Pressure-induced fast axonal transport abnormalities and the anatomy at the lamina cribrosa in primate eyes. Invest Ophthalmol Vis Sci 1983; 24:343–346.
19. Morgan JE. Selective cell death in glaucoma: does it really occur? Br J Ophthalmol 1994; 78:875–879.
20. Campbell FW, Maffei L. Contrast and spatial frequency. Sci Am 1974; 231:106–114.
21. Campbell FW, Robson JG. Application of Fourier analysis to the visibility of gratings. J Physiol 1968; 197:551–566.
22. Arden G. Measuring contrast sensitivity with gratings: A new simple technique for the early diagnosis of retinal and neurological disease. J Am Optom Assoc 1979; 50:35–39.
23. Atkin A, Bodis-Wollner I, Wolkstein M, et al. Abnormalities of central contrast sensitivity in glaucoma. Am J Ophthalmol 1979; 88:205–211.
24. Bron AJ. Contrast sensitivity changes in ocular hypertension and early glaucoma. Surv Ophthalmol 1989; 33 Suppl:405–406.

25. Hawkins AS, Szlyk JP, Ardickas Z, et al. Comparison of contrast sensitivity, visual acuity, and Humphrey visual field testing in patients with glaucoma. J Glaucoma 2003; 12:134–138.

26. Korth M, Horn F, Storck B, et al. Spatial and spatiotemporal contrast sensitivity of normal and glaucoma eyes. Graefes Arch Clin Exp Ophthalmol 1989; 227:428–435.

27. Lundh BL. Central contrast sensitivity tests in the detection of early glaucoma. Acta Ophthalmol (Copenh) 1985; 63:481–486.

28. Ross JE. Clinical detection of abnormalities in central vision in chronic simple glaucoma using contrast sensitivity. Int Ophthalmol 1985; 8:167–177.

29. Ross JE, Bron AJ, Clarke DD. Contrast sensitivity and visual disability in chronic simple glaucoma. Br J Ophthalmol 1984, 68:821 827.

30. Sample PA, Juang PS, Weinreb RN. Isolating the effects of primary open-angle glaucoma on the contrast sensitivity function. Am J Ophthalmol 1991; 112:308–316.

31. Wood JM, Lovie-Kitchin JE. Evaluation of the efficacy of contrast sensitivity measures for the detection of early primary open-angle glaucoma. Optom Vis Sci 1992; 69;175–181.

32. Breton ME, Wilson TW, Wilson R, et al. Temporal contrast sensitivity loss in primary open-angle glaucoma and glaucoma suspects. Invest Ophthalmol Vis Sci 1991; 32:2931–2941.

33. Brussell EM, White CW, Faubert J, et al. Multiflash campimetry as an indicator of visual field loss in glaucoma. Am J Optom Physiol Opt 1986; 63:32–40.

34. Holopigian K, Seiple W, Mayron C, et al. Electrophysiological and psychophysical flicker sensitivity in patients with primary open-angle glaucoma and ocular hypertension. Invest Ophthalmol Vis Sci 1990; 31:1863–1868.

35. Adams AJ, Heron G, Husted R. Clinical measures of central vision function in glaucoma and ocular hypertension. Arch Ophthalmol 1987; 105:782–787.

36. Adams AJ, Rodic R, Husted R, et al. Spectral sensitivity and color discrimination changes in glaucoma and glaucoma-suspect patients. Invest Ophthalmol Vis Sci 1982; 23:516–524.

37. Austin DJ. Acquired colour vision defects in patients suffering from chronic simple glaucoma. Trans Ophthalmol Soc UK 1974; 94:880–883.

38. Drance SM, Lakowski R, Schulzer M, et al. Acquired color vision changes in glaucoma. Use of 100-hue test and Pickford anomaloscope as predictors of glaucomatous field change. Arch Ophthalmol 1981; 99:829–831.

39. Flammer J, Drance SM. Correlation between color vision scores and quantitative perimetry in suspected glaucoma. Arch Ophthalmol 1984; 102:38 39.

40. Grutzner P, Schleicher S. Acquired color vision defects in glaucoma patients. Mod Probl Ophthalmol 1972; 11:136–140.

41. Gunduz K, Arden GB, Perry S, et al. Color vision defects in ocular hypertension and glaucoma. Quantification with a computer-driven color television system. Arch Ophthalmol 1988; 106:929–935.

42. Kelly JP, Fourman SM, Jindra LF. Foveal color and luminance sensitivity losses in glaucoma. Ophthalmic Surg Lasers 1996; 27:179–187.

43. Lakowski R, Bryett J, Drance SM. A study of colour vision in ocular hypertensives. Can J Ophthalmol 1972; 7:86–95.

44. Poinoosawmy D, Nagasubramanian S, Gloster J. Colour vision in patients with chronic simple glaucoma and ocular hypertension. Br J Ophthalmol 1980; 64:852–857.

45. Yamazaki Y, Lakowski R, Drance SM. A comparison of the blue color mechanism in high- and low-tension glaucoma. Ophthalmology 1989; 96:12–15.

46. Drance SM. The glaucomatous visual field. Br J Ophthalmol 1972; 56:186–200.

47. de Jong LA, Snepvangers CE, van den Berg TJ, et al. Blue-yellow perimetry in the detection of early glaucomatous damage. Doc Ophthalmol 1990; 75:303–314.

48. Heron G, Adams AJ, Husted R. Foveal and non-foveal measures of short wavelength sensitive pathways in glaucoma and ocular hypertension. Ophthalmic Physiol Opt 1987; 7.403–404.

49. Teesalu P. Blue-on-yellow perimetry in the diagnosis of glaucoma. Acta Ophthalmol Scand 1999; 77:364–365.

50. Wild JM. Short wavelength automated perimetry. Acta Ophthalmol Scand 2001; 79:546–559.

51. Wild JM, Moss ID, Whitaker D, et al. The statistical interpretation of blue-on-yellow visual field loss. Invest Ophthalmol Vis Sci 1995; 36:1398–1410.

52. Horn F, Martus P, Korth M. Comparison of temporal and spatiotemporal contrast-sensitivity

tests in normal subjects and glaucoma patients. Ger J Ophthalmol 1995; 4:97–102.

53. Horn FK, Jonas JB, Korth M, et al. The full-field flicker test in early diagnosis of chronic open-angle glaucoma. Am J Ophthalmol 1997; 123:313–319.

54. Horn FK, Velten IM, Junemann A, et al. The full-field flicker test in glaucomas: influence of intraocular pressure and pattern of visual field losses. Graefes Arch Clin Exp Ophthalmol 1999; 237:621–628.

55. Velten IM, Korth M, Horn FK, et al. Temporal contrast sensitivity with peripheral and central stimulation in glaucoma diagnosis. Br J Ophthalmol 1999; 83:199–205.

56. Lachenmayr BJ. The role of temporal threshold criteria in psychophysical testing in glaucoma. Curr Opin Ophthalmol 1994; 5:58–63.

57. Lachenmayr BJ, Drance SM, Douglas GR, et al. Light-sense, flicker and resolution perimetry in glaucoma: a comparative study. Graefes Arch Clin Exp Ophthalmol 1991; 229:246–251.

58. Lachenmayr BJ, Kojetinsky S, Ostermaier N, et al. The different effects of aging on normal sensitivity in flicker and light-sense perimetry. Invest Ophthalmol Vis Sci 1994; 35:2741–2748.

59. Lachenmayr BJ, Gleissner M. Flicker perimetry resists retinal image degradation. Invest Ophthalmol Vis Sci 1992; 33:3539–3542.

60. Kelly DH. Nonlinear visual responses to flickering sinusoidal gratings. J Opt Soc Am 1981; 71:1051–1055.

61. Johnson CA, Samuels SJ. Screening for glaucomatous visual field loss with frequency-doubling perimetry. Invest Ophthalmol Vis Sci 1997; 38:413–425.

62. Johnson CA, Cioffi GA, Van Buskirk EM. Frequency doubling technology perimetry using a 24–2 stimulus presentation pattern. Optom Vis Sci 1999; 76:571–581.

63. Alward WL. Frequency doubling technology perimetry for the detection of glaucomatous visual field loss. Am J Ophthalmol 2000; 129:376–378.

64. Brusini P, Busatto P. Frequency doubling perimetry in glaucoma early diagnosis. Acta Ophthalmol Scand Suppl 1998; (227):23–4.

65. Cagigrigoriu A, Rabbione MM, Onnis E, et al. Comparison between results obtained with traditional perimetry and those with frequency doubling perimetry in initial phase chronic simple glaucoma. Acta Ophthalmol Scand Suppl 2000; (232):24–26.

66. Maddess T, Severt WL, Stange G. Comparison of three tests using the frequency doubling illusion to diagnose glaucoma. Clin Experiment Ophthalmol 2001; 29:359–367.

67. Quigley HA. Identification of glaucoma-related visual field abnormality with the screening protocol of frequency doubling technology. Am J Ophthalmol 1998; 125:819–829.

68. Serguhn S, Spiegel D. Comparison of frequency doubling perimetry and standard achromatic computerized perimetry in patients with glaucoma. Graefes Arch Clin Exp Ophthalmol 2001; 239:351–355.

69. Thomas R, Bhat S, Muliyil JP, et al. Frequency doubling perimetry in glaucoma. J Glaucoma 2002; 11:46–50.

70. Shabana N, Peres VC, Carkeet A, et al. Motion perception in glaucoma patients: a review. Surv Ophthalmol 2003; 48:92–106.

71. Baez KA, McNaught AI, Dowler JG, et al. Motion detection threshold and field progression in normal tension glaucoma. Br J Ophthalmol 1995; 79:125–128.

72. Bosworth CF, Sample PA, Gupta N, et al. Motion automated perimetry identifies early glaucomatous field defects. Arch Ophthalmol 1998; 116:1153–1158.

73. Bullimore MA, Wood JM, Swenson K. Motion perception in glaucoma. Invest Ophthalmol Vis Sci 1993; 34:3526–3533.

74. Silverman SE, Trick GL, Hart WM, Jr. Motion perception is abnormal in primary open-angle glaucoma and ocular hypertension. Invest Ophthalmol Vis Sci 1990; 31:722–729.

75. Trick GL, Steinman SB, Amyot M. Motion perception deficits in glaucomatous optic neuropathy. Vision Res 1995; 35:2225–2233.

76. Wu J, Coffey M, Reidy A, et al. Impaired motion sensitivity as a predictor of subsequent field loss in glaucoma suspects: the Roscommon Glaucoma Study. Br J Ophthalmol 1998; 82:534–537.

77. Sahraie A, Barbur JL, Edgar DF, et al. Motion discrimination of single targets: comparison of preliminary findings in normal subjects and patients with glaucoma. Graefes Arch Clin Exp Ophthalmol 1996; 234:553–560.

78. Westcott MC, Fitzke FW, Hitchings RA. Abnormal motion displacement thresholds are associated with fine scale luminance sensitivity loss in glaucoma. Vision Res 1998; 38:3171–3180.

79. Frisen L. High-pass resolution perimetry. A clinical review. Doc Ophthalmol 1993; 83:1–25.

80. Chauhan BC, House PH, McCormick TA, et al. Comparison of conventional and high-pass resolution perimetry in a prospective study of patients with glaucoma and healthy controls. Arch Ophthalmol 1999; 117:24–33.

81. Chauhan BC. The value of high-pass resolution perimetry in glaucoma. Curr Opin Ophthalmol 2000; 11:85–89.

82. Iester M, Capris P, Altieri M, et al. Correlation between high-pass resolution perimetry and standard threshold perimetry in subjects with glaucoma and ocular hypertension. Int Ophthalmol 1999; 23:99–103.

83. Kono Y, Chi QM, Tomita G, et al. High-pass resolution perimetry and a Humphrey Field Analyzer as indicators of glaucomatous optic disc abnormalities. A comparative study. Ophthalmology 1997; 104:1496–1502.

84. Martinez GA, Sample PA, Weinreb RN. Comparison of high-pass resolution perimetry and standard automated perimetry in glaucoma. Am J Ophthalmol 1995; 119:195–201.

85. Sample PA, Ahn DS, Lee PC, et al. High-pass resolution perimetry in eyes with ocular hypertension and primary open-angle glaucoma. Am J Ophthalmol 1992; 113:309–316.

86. Tomita G, Maeda M, Sogano S, et al. An analysis of the relationship between high-pass resolution perimetry and neuroretinal rim area in normal-tension glaucoma. Acta Ophthalmol (Copenh) 1993; 71:196–200.

87. Drum B, Breton M, Massof R. Pattern discrimination perimetry: A new concept in visual field testing. In: Greve EL, Heijl A, eds. Seventh International Visual Field Symposium. The Netherlands: Kluwer Academic Publishers; 1986:433–440.

88. Ansari I, Chauhan BC, McCormick TA, et al. Comparison of conventional and pattern discrimination perimetry in a prospective study of glaucoma patients. Invest Ophthalmol Vis Sci 2000; 41:4150–4157.

89. Chauhan BC, LeBlanc RP, McCormick TA, et al. Comparison of high-pass resolution perimetry and pattern discrimination perimetry to conventional perimetry in glaucoma. Can J Ophthalmol 1993; 28:306–311.

90. Chauhan BC, LeBlanc RP, McCormick TA, et al. Correlation between the optic disc and results obtained with conventional, high-pass resolution and pattern discrimination perimetry in glaucoma. Can J Ophthalmol 1993; 28:312–316.

91. Nutaitis MJ, Stewart WC, Kelly DM, et al. Pattern discrimination perimetry in patients with glaucoma and ocular hypertension. Am J Ophthalmol 1992; 114:297–301.

92. Stewart WC, Connor AB, Rogers GM. Correlation of pattern discrimination perimetry to the optic disc and visual field in ocular hypertensive and chronic open-angle glaucoma patients. Int Ophthalmol 1995; 19:101–107.

93. Riggs LA, Johnson EP, Schick AML. Electrical responses of the human eye to changes in wavelength. J Opt Soc Am 1966; 56:1621–1627.

94. Maffei L, Fiorentini A. Electroretinographic responses to alternating gratings in the cat. Exp Brain Res 1982; 48:327–334.

95. Maffei L, Fiorentini A, Bisti S, et al. Pattern ERG in the monkey after section of the optic nerve. Exp Brain Res 1985; 59:423–425.

96. Arai M, Yoshimura N, Sakaue H, et al. A 3-year follow-up study of ocular hypertension by pattern electroretinogram. Ophthalmologica 1993; 207:187–195.

97. Bach M, Speidel-Fiaux A. Pattern electroretinogram in glaucoma and ocular hypertension. Doc Ophthalmol 1989; 73:173–181.

98. Garway-Heath DF, Holder GE, Fitzke FW, et al. Relationship between electrophysiological, psychophysical, and anatomical measurements in glaucoma. Invest Ophthalmol Vis Sci 2002; 43:2213–2220.

99. Hull BM, Thompson DA. A review of the clinical applications of the pattern electroretinogram. Ophthalmic Physiol Opt 1989; 9:143–152.

100. Marx MS, Podos SM, Bodis-Wollner I, et al. Signs of early damage in glaucomatous monkey eyes: low spatial frequency losses in the pattern ERG and VEP. Exp Eye Res 1988; 46:173–184.

101. Pfeiffer N, Tillmon B, Bach M. Predictive value of the pattern electroretinogram in high-risk ocular hypertension. Invest Ophthalmol Vis Sci 1993; 34:1710–1715.

102. Pfeiffer N, Bach M. The pattern-electroretinogram in glaucoma and ocular hypertension. A cross-sectional and longitudinal study. Ger J Ophthalmol 1992; 1:35–40.

103. Rimmer S, Katz B. The pattern electroretinogram: technical aspects and clinical significance. J Clin Neurophysiol 1989; 6:85–99.

104. van den Berg TJ, Riemslag FC, de Vos GW, et al. Pattern ERG and glaucomatous visual field defects. Doc Ophthalmol 1986; 61:335–341.

105. Vitale BF, Brogliatti B, Fea A, et al. Sector PERG evaluation of glaucomatous damage. Acta Ophthalmol Scand Suppl 1997; 50–1.

Chapter 7

Diagnosis of the glaucomas 1: visual field changes

David B Henson and Robert Harper

7.1 INTRODUCTION

The role of visual field measurement in the shared care of primary open angle glaucoma (POAG) can be broadly divided into two parts: the detection of visual field loss in an eye which formerly had no visual field loss and the detection of progressive loss in an eye with established loss.

The detection of visual field loss and the detection of change are two very different problems and for this reason this chapter is divided into two main sections. The first section briefly presents a classification of visual field loss seen in POAG and their evolution, before going on to discuss the techniques used to establish whether or not a visual field defect exists. The second section deals with the monitoring of glaucomatous visual field loss and the techniques which have been developed to establish whether or not the visual field defect has changed.

7.2 DETECTING VISUAL FIELD LOSS IN POAG

7.2.1 VISUAL FIELD DEFECTS ASSOCIATED WITH POAG

Visual field defects associated with POAG are as follows:

- Paracentral defects
- Arcuate defects
- Nasal step

- Overall depression in sensitivity
- Baring of the blind spot
- Enlargement of the blind spot.

Chapter 5 describes and illustrates the above visual field defects. The first three are collectively known as nerve fibre bundle defects and are highly specific to glaucoma (good discriminatory power). The last three are often seen in other pathologies and are, therefore, less useful when trying to detect glaucoma. Although overall depression is reported to occur in a significant percentage of cases,[1] it is not specific to POAG. Cataracts can cause a similar overall depression, as do the normally occurring age changes in the retina. Henson et al[2] questioned whether generalised depression does actually occur across the whole visual field. Using a full threshold technique in a group of normal and glaucomatous eyes (with early field loss), they established that even at the most sensitive locations of the visual field, locations that were well away from any localised loss, the glaucomatous eyes had a lower sensitivity than the normal ones of between 1 dB and 2 dB. They concluded that purely localised loss is a rare event although the extent of the diffuse loss is often slight and difficult to establish within a clinical situation.

7.2.2 EVOLUTION OF GLAUCOMATOUS FIELD DEFECTS

The earliest sign of glaucomatous loss is an increased variability of responses in an area which subsequently develops a repeatable defect.[3] This can manifest itself as a patient missing a stimulus and then seeing it when represented. Defects then enlarge and deepen but are often confined to either the superior or inferior field. In some patients an entire hemifield may be lost before the second hemifield becomes involved.

While POAG is invariably a bilateral condition (involving both the right and left eyes), its progression is often asymmetrical, occurring in one eye before the other and, when both eyes are involved, being more advanced in one eye compared with the other. The recognition of this asymmetry, which has been reported to occur in over 90% of glaucomatous cases, is useful in the early diagnosis of POAG. In addition to the asymmetries between the two eyes, there is frequently an asymmetry between the superior and inferior hemifields. STATPAC 2 uses this type of asymmetry to help identify patients with glaucomatous visual field loss.[4]

7.2.3 METHODS FOR DETECTING VISUAL FIELD LOSS

One of the simplest ways of detecting visual field loss is via visual inspection, which can take into account a host of parameters including:

- Location of defect
- Artefacts, such as those caused by the correcting lens rim
- Right/left eye asymmetry
- Superior/inferior hemifield asymmetry.

One of the problems with visual inspection is the lack of clearly defined criteria. What one clinician will view as a significant visual field defect does not necessarily equate with the view of another clinician. A slightly more sophisticated way of defining visual field loss is to augment visual inspection with a series of rules. There are many different sets but a typical set might be: three or more contiguous non-edge points that on full threshold perimetry are depressed by at least 5 dB from their average age-specific normal threshold values. At least one of the points has to be depressed by 10 dB. These rules, while helping to overcome the criticism levelled above, have rarely been subjected to population studies in which their specificity and sensitivity have been evaluated.

A better way of defining visual field loss is to quantify the results and then compare the value(s) with those from a normal population. This approach has been used for both full threshold and suprathreshold perimetry. With full threshold perimetry the global indices *mean defect, mean deviation, loss variance, pattern standard deviation* etc. (see Chapter 5) have all been used, as have scoring systems based upon the number and location of depressed points.[5] With suprathreshold perimetry, Henson and Bryson developed a scoring system which took into account the number, depth and cluster properties of the missed stimuli.[6] The result was presented on a probability scale divided into three regions—normal, suspect and defect—

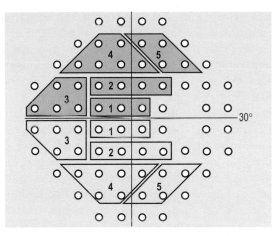

Fig. 7.1 Zones used in the Humphrey Visual Field Analyzer's Glaucoma Hemifield Test. (Reproduced from Heijl A, Lindgren G, Lindgren A, et al[4] with permission from the publisher.)

the normal/suspect border being at the 10% probability level and the suspect/defect border being at the 0.1% level. (Tests based upon comparing the results of a scoring system to a normal population are establishing whether or not the result comes from a 'normal' eye rather than establishing whether or not the eye is glaucomatous.)

The use of scoring systems has been further developed by Heijl et al who introduced the Glaucoma Hemifield Test (GHT).[4] This test uses asymmetry between the superior and inferior hemifields to establish whether or not a defect exists. Each hemifield is divided into five mirror-image sectors on the basis of the nerve fibre distribution (Fig. 7.1). Pattern deviation probability values for each test location are used to derive a score for each sector. By comparing the score for each sector with that from its mirror image in the other hemifield, and then comparing the results to those from a normal population, Heijl et al[4] were able to establish the likelihood of the result arising from a 'normal' eye. Their method, while using a scoring system, classifies each visual field result into one of five groups (within normal limits, borderline, outside normal limits, general reduction in sensitivity and abnormally high sensitivity).

Many of the scoring systems described above are sensitive to the existence of artefacts, such as those produced by the rims of correcting lenses. Those based on suprathreshold perimetry are also sensitive to an error in the thresholding phase of the examination. If the thresholding phase sets the test intensity too close to the threshold then there is a danger that patients without significant visual field loss will be classified as beyond the normal limit.

In Section 7.2 it was pointed out that the earliest visual field defect seen in POAG was an increase in the variability in and around an area which subsequently goes on to develop a repeatable visual field defect. This increase in variability can result in transient visual field defects, ones which are present at one visit but disappear at the next. Heijl and Bengtsson have shown that transient defects can occur for periods ranging from 1 to 6 years (average 3.5).[3] This finding has important implications for shared care schemes. Should the shared care practitioner re-refer the patient as soon as they get an abnormal finding or should they wait until the abnormal finding is repeatable? In the first instance they run the risk of generating what might well be a false positive, while in the second situation they run the risk of deferring treatment until significant damage has occurred.

Notwithstanding the limitations imposed by the transient nature of early visual field loss, the scoring techniques described above give a sensitive and specific measure of the presence of visual field loss. This is due to the fact that patients with normal visual fields show little variability. As will be shown in section 7.3, this is not the case when we come to look at the results from patients with glaucomatous field loss.

7.3 DETECTING CHANGE IN A DEFECTIVE VISUAL FIELD

For many years the successful treatment of POAG has been seen as achieving a 'target pressure'. This concept has a number of shortcomings, the major one being that intraocular pressure (IOP) is a risk factor and not a measure of visual function, the retention of which is the main objective of treatment. Recently the emphasis of successful treatment has shifted towards looking at visual outcomes.[7] To predict long-term visual outcomes the clinician needs to know what the current rate of visual field loss is and then relate this to the patient's life expectancy. Clearly, an acceptable rate of loss, which is arguably one which does not result in any significant visual disability throughout the remainder of the patient's life, is dependent upon the patient's age. In a young person a very slow rate of change may ultimately lead to severe visual disability, whereas a more rapid rate of loss in an elderly patient may have little, if any, effect upon the patient's long-term quality of life.

Inherent within the objective to retain quality of life is the need to measure accurately the rate of visual field loss and the extent to which this rate is affected by different therapeutic measures. This need has spurred a great deal of ophthalmic research, which forms the bulk of the information presented below. Being able to discriminate change in the visual field from noise is the crux of the problem, and the following section describes variability and the parameters which are known to affect it. This is followed by a description of the major quantification systems which have been introduced to assist the clinician in recognising change, and by a section on the classification and grading of visual field defects. Finally, a number of practical points are presented to help practitioners decide whether or not the visual field has changed since the last visit.

7.3.1 VARIABILITY

Figure 7.2 gives the results from a Humphrey Visual Field Analyzer (HFA) 24-2 test carried out on a patient with a superior hemifield loss. The defect is clearly seen in the gray scale plot of threshold values at the top right-hand side of the figure. At the top left are the raw threshold data for each tested location. It can be seen that low threshold values correspond to the dark areas on the gray scale. The 24-2 programme of the HFA instrument tests some locations twice. When a repeat measurement is made the second threshold estimate is printed, in brackets, below the first. By looking at the repeat measures we can estimate how variable the results are. What we would like to see is no difference between the initial and repeat values. Looking at the repeat values in the inferior

visual field of Fig. 7.2—where the thresholds are near normal—we can see that while the repeat measures may differ by a few decibels there are no major differences between the initial and repeat values. When we look at the results in the superior visual field, especially towards the edge of the defective region, there are occasions when large differences exist between the two threshold estimates. In some cases the sensitivity gets worse on the repeat measurement, whereas in others it gets better. It is important to remember that the results given in Fig. 7.2 have all been obtained within a single session and that the algorithm used to collect the data randomises the order of presentations. The increase in variability is not, therefore, simply due to the timing of the presentations.

This example highlights the finding by Werner and Drance,[8] that variability increases in areas of the visual field which have been damaged by POAG, since confirmed by a large number of researchers including Henson et al.[9] This increase in variability is not specific to a particular instrument or to a particular strategy or in fact to glaucoma. It has, however, a major impact on our ability to differentiate between progressive loss and noise.

Some of the best research on variability in glaucoma has not used repeat measures but frequency-of-seeing (FOS) curves. These curves, which plot the relation between the frequency of a seen response and stimulus intensity, give a precise measure of threshold sensitivity and variability. In a FOS curve the threshold is normally taken as the intensity at which 50% of the stimuli are seen, and the gradient of the FOS curve is a measure of variability. Some examples of FOS curves are given in Fig. 7.3 for both normal and glaucomatous eyes. In glaucoma, visual field regions of near normal sensitivity give similar responses to those from normal eyes, while regions where the sensitivity is depressed give much shallower gradients (increased variability). The relationship between threshold sensitivity and gradient of the FOS curve has been described by a number of researchers.[9,10] Figure 7.4 gives the results from Weber and Rau,[10] which show a very tight relationship between variability and sensitivity. This relationship not only holds for glaucomatous eyes but also for central and peripheral test locations in normal eyes, i.e. in

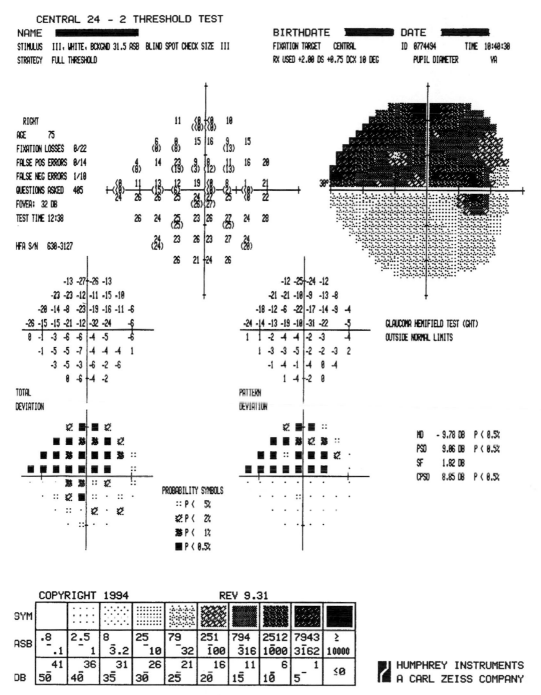

Fig. 7.2 Result from a full threshold (24-2) test on a Humphrey Visual Field Analyzer. The patient has superior hemifield loss.

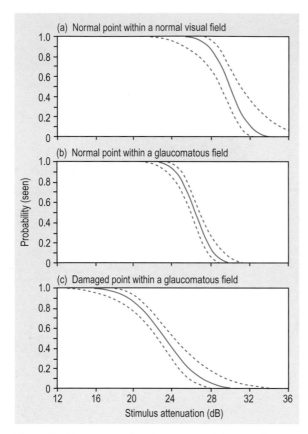

Fig. 7.3 Frequency of seeing curves. (**a**) Normal location in a normal visual field.
(**b**) Normal location in a patient with glaucomatous visual field loss.
(**c**) Defective location in a patient with glaucomatous visual field loss.

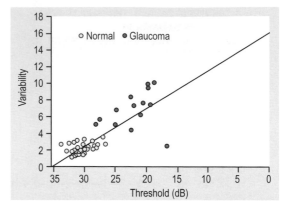

Fig. 7.4 Relationship between the gradient of the frequency of seeing curve and threshold. (Redrawn from Weber and Rau[10] with permission from the publisher.)

a normal eye the sensitivity in the peripheral field is less than that at the centre and the variability is greater.

Several theories have been proposed to explain the increase in variability seen in and around areas of glaucomatous damage. One theory, the reduced redundancy theory, is based upon the density of ganglion cells. This theory assumes that isolated ganglion cells give variable (noisy) responses, however, the pooled response from a large number of ganglion cells is relatively constant. In the normal eye the standard white-on-white, 0.43° diameter stimulus falls upon a fairly large number of ganglion cells and the responses are, therefore, fairly constant (low variability). As the number of

ganglion cells is reduced, either by moving into the peripheral visual field or through pathological damage, so the inherent variability of individual ganglion cells becomes more apparent. Support for this theory comes from a large number of research findings including:

- The relationship of variability to stimulus size, with large stimuli giving less variability than small stimuli.
- The increase in variability with target eccentricity as the density of ganglion cells is reduced.
- The increase in variability around the blind spot where the density of ganglion cells is reduced.
- The increase in variability with blue on yellow perimetry, which selectively tests a smaller population of ganglion cells.
- The increase in variability found in other pathologies which reduce the number of ganglion cells.

Whatever the cause of the increased variability seen in areas of glaucomatous damage, its effect is to hinder the accurate measurement of both the visual field and the rate of visual field loss. To obtain reliable estimates of the rate of loss it is currently necessary to have a large number of visual field results, placing a considerable burden on healthcare resources.

The localised nature of the increase in variability seen in POAG brings into question the concept of global measures of variability. The visual field indices, fluctuation, corrected loss variance and corrected pattern standard deviation (see Chapter 5 section 5.7.3), all make the assumption that variability within a visual field can be represented by a single number. The data presented above demonstrate that this assumption is not valid and the global measure of variability—fluctuation—is an out-of-date concept.

7.3.2 DETECTING CHANGE IN THE VISUAL FIELD

One of the most widely used techniques for detecting change in the visual field is visual inspection and comparison of the visual field charts. This technique can take into account a whole series of parameters including:

■ Changes in the area, depth and number of defects
■ Whether or not the defects are close to the macula
■ Artefacts, such as those produced by the correcting lens rim
■ Reliability estimates
■ The results from the other eye.

Visual inspection can be applied to any number of visual field charts and can, within limits, be used to combine data from different instruments/strategies. It is important to remember that many of the parameters taken into account by the experienced clinician are ignored by even the most sophisticated analytical techniques (see below). For example analytical techniques rarely take into account the spatial pattern of loss, e.g. they cannot differentiate between a lens rim artefact and an arcuate scotoma. The sudden occurrence of a lens rim artefact can, therefore, often be misinterpreted by these analytical systems as a sign of progression. It is only when the clinician views the respective visual field charts that the true status is established. There are, however, a number of problems with visual inspection:

■ The clinician is often presented with such a large amount of data that it is difficult to 'take it all in'.
■ A belief that analytical techniques may be more sensitive to change, signalling significant progression at an earlier stage when less damage has occurred.

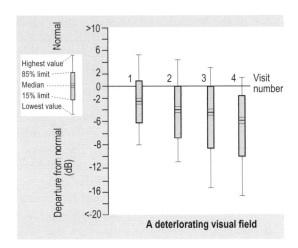

Fig. 7.5 Box and whisker plot showing a deteriorating visual field in a patient with glaucoma.

■ Visual inspection cannot give the precise measures of progression needed for the long-term prediction of visual outcomes.

There are several graphical techniques available to overcome the first problem. Some simply reproduce, on a single sheet, a subset of the data given in a series of visual field charts, e.g. the HFA Overview Printout. This makes it easier for the clinician to recognise trends and the degree of variability in the data. Others present the data in a different format, e.g. the box and whisker plot.

Box and whisker plots

Box and whisker plots are used in statistics to represent distributions. They can take on a variety of forms, representing parameters such as the mean, median, standard deviation, confidence limits, percentile limits, maximum and minimum values. The STATPAC 2 analysis of the HFA uses box and whisker plots to present the age-corrected deviation values of each visual field response[4] (Fig. 7.5). The box gives the median (dark line) and the 15 and 85 percentile responses (top and bottom of the box) while the whiskers give the worst and best responses. The value of this data reduction technique is highlighted in Fig. 7.5 where the results from several visual field examinations can be seen at a glance.

One of the first attempts to statistically evaluate whether or not the visual field had changed was developed for the Octopus instrument and incorporated in their Delta software package.[11] This test compared the sensitivity, at each test location, of two records and computed the mean difference and the distribution of the differences. If there is no change in the visual field then the mean difference should be close to zero. The t test is used to establish the significance of any change. Hills and Johnson evaluated this method of detecting visual field changes.[12] They used real visual field records into which they inserted a scotoma of known depth and size and then computed how this would affect the t test values. They found that although the test was very sensitive to small changes in the entire visual field it was relatively insensitive to scotoma <18° in diameter, even when the sensitivity loss was as great as 35 dB. They concluded that this statistical test had limited ability to detect clinically significant change, and was further limited by the fact that it can only be applied to two sets of data. When more than two sets are available the intermediate sets are either ignored or averaged with the other sets.

Linear regression

The limitation of only being able to evaluate the change between two sets of data was overcome by the use of linear regression.[13] Linear regression is incorporated in the STATPAC 2 analysis of the HFA where the global index *mean deviation* is regressed over time (this analysis is only performed if five or more test results are available). Data is presented in the form of the rate of visual field loss in dB/year and its 95% confidence limits. From these values the clinician can estimate the long-term visual outcomes for the patient. Some of the problems associated with making predictions from this type of data are highlighted in Fig. 7.6. In Fig. 7.6a there are five visual field records taken over a 2.5-year period in a patient who was first seen at the age of 60 years. The measures show some variability, typical of that found in a glaucoma patient. A linear regression analysis has been performed which predicts that the patient will have no visual field when they reach 72 years of age. Also shown

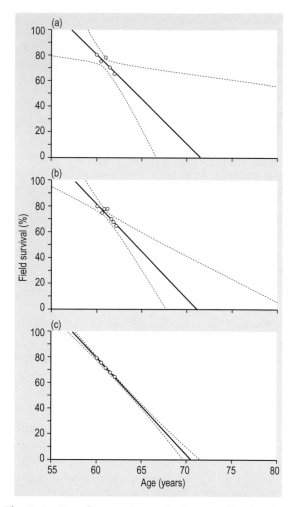

Fig. 7.6 Use of regression analysis to predict visual field survival in a patient. The bold solid lines are the best fitting (least squares) fit to the data and the dotted lines represent the 95% confidence limits. (**a**) Best fitting line to 5 sets of data recorded at 6 month intervals. Note the wide confidence limits. (**b**) The addition of two extra measurements (seven in all) improves the fit, i.e. reduces the spread of the confidence limits. (**c**) Reducing the variability of the data greatly improves the quality of the fit and allows accurate prediction of long-term field survival.

on the graph are the 95% confidence limits for the prediction. These limits show that the patient may go blind when they reach 67 years of age or that they may never go blind. The wide confidence limits are a reflection of the variability in the data and the limited number of visual field records. Increasing the number of records in the analysis, as shown in Fig. 7.6b, reduces the spread of the 95% confidence limits and improves the accuracy of the prediction. However, reducing the variability in the data has a much greater effect on the confidence limits (Fig. 7.6c). In this example, when variability is reduced, we can make a much more accurate prediction, i.e. that the patient will lose all their visual field when they get to between 69 and 72 years of age. This example highlights the importance of developing visual field indices which tackle the problem of variability.

The regression analysis used in the HFA pools the data from the whole visual field. Werner et al[11] and O'Brien and Schwartz[14] reported that when linear regression was applied to different sectors of the visual field the performance of this type of analysis improved. They found several cases where a significant change could be detected with sector analysis which would have been missed by a global analysis. The process of performing regression analysis on areas of the visual field rather than on the whole visual field was taken a stage further by Noureddin et al[15] and Wild et al[16] who regressed each test location over time. This pointwise analysis is also used in the software package Progressor,[17] which employs a novel technique to display the results of the analysis superimposed upon the visual field chart (Fig. 7.7). This technique allows the clinician to see not only which locations are progressing, but also the spatial relations of the progressing locations. Viswanathan et al[18] have demonstrated how this technique is superior to that currently used in STATPAC 2 at detecting progressive loss. The latest version of the software provides an estimate of the rate of loss both globally and at individual locations.

A major limitation of regression analysis is the need for large amounts of visual field data, e.g. the STATPAC 2 analysis requires a minimum of five visual field tests before it will generate an estimate of the rate of loss. Clinicians often want to know whether or not a medical or surgical change introduced at the last examination has arrested the progression of field loss, and are understandably reluctant to wait until a further five sets of data have been collected. STATPAC 2 also introduced

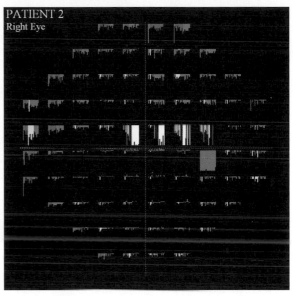

Fig. 7.7 Output from the software package Progressor. (Reproduced with permission of Mr A Viswanathan, Moorfields Eye Hospital NHSFT, London.)

'Glaucoma Change Probability Analysis' to try to overcome this problem.[4] This analysis establishes whether or not there has been any significant progression at each test location from a baseline of two or three earlier visual field records. The analysis uses a reference database collected from both normal and glaucomatous eyes which empirically corrects for the increased variability seen in POAG.

The above discussion has addressed the monitoring of change with full threshold perimetry. Relatively little research has been published on the use of alternative strategies to monitor glaucomatous visual field loss. The Bristol Shared Care Glaucoma Study monitored POAG with suprathreshold perimetry.[19] This study used the results from an unpublished trial of 174 glaucomatous eyes (monitored for 2 years) to calculate the change in the number of missed stimuli from one visit to the next and the confidence limits for the change. The Bristol study used a two-stage criterion for the detection of progression: in the first stage, if a patient misses an additional seven or more stimuli (all practitioners used a 132-point central test strategy on a Henson perimeter) they are booked in for a second visual field test within the next 2 weeks.

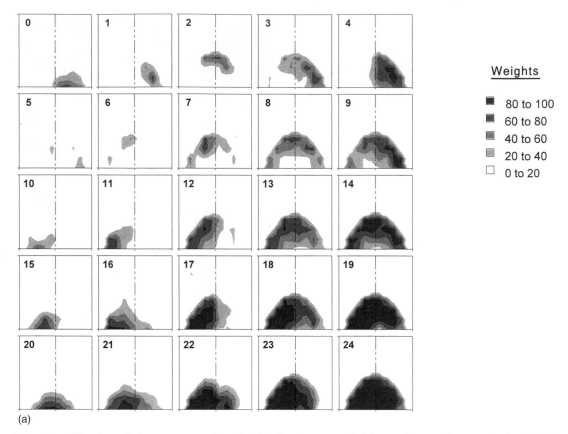

(a)

Fig. 7.8a Classification of glaucomatous visual field defect by an artificial neural network: superior hemifield classification.

If, when the results of the two tests are averaged, the patient is missing four or more additional stimuli then they are classified as progressing.

Later work, based upon the results from the Bristol study,[20] has demonstrated improved ability to detect change if the superior and inferior hemifields are analysed separately and the depth of the defects is taken into account.

7.3.3 CLASSIFICATION OF DEFECTS: GRADING VISUAL FIELD LOSS

A completely different way of establishing whether or not there has been a change in the visual field is to classify each visual field defect and to see whether or not there has been a change in the classification. Aulhorn and Harms classified the visual fields of 954 eyes with glaucomatous loss into eight different groups.[21] The subjective classification was based upon the location, shape and extent of loss. Similar descriptive classifications have been given by Drance,[22] and as part of an investigation into progressive loss by both Hart and Becker[23] and Jay and Murdoch.[24] These subjective classification systems have too few classes for the monitoring of individual cases.

This problem has been overcome through the use of artificial neural networks (ANNs). Henson et al used a self-organising feature map to spatially classify the types of visual field defect seen in glaucoma.[25] They chose to separately analyse the superior and inferior hemifields and to configure the ANN to produce 25 different classes of superior and inferior loss (Fig. 7.8). An important characteristic of the ANN used in this research was that the individual classes form a continuum across the map, i.e. as a patient's visual field loss progresses the defects gradually move across the map from the earliest defect, normally in or close to one corner, to the most advanced defect in the opposite corner.

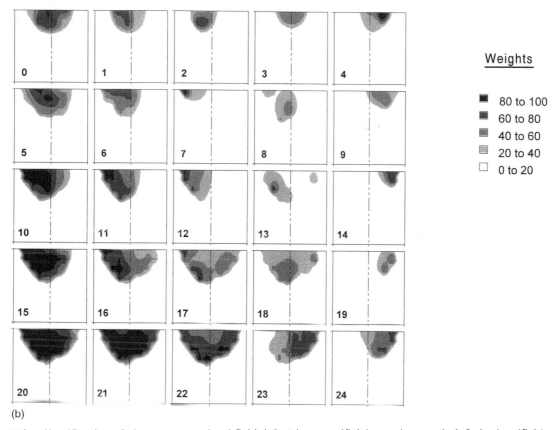

(b)

Fig. 7.8b Classification of glaucomatous visual field defect by an artificial neural network: inferior hemifield classification.

The ANN classification system has many advantages over the previously described classification systems:

- The classification is not based upon any preconceived ideas about the nature of glaucomatous visual field loss.
- It can be used to give a finer classification (more classes) which improves its potential for monitoring visual field loss.
- It is not confused by the occurrence of defects which appear to lie at boundaries between one class and another or by defects which appear to have the characteristics of more than one class.

While the use of ANNs to monitor glaucomatous loss is certainly an attractive route to follow it does not overcome the problems associated with variability, because noisy visual field data will result in noisy spatial classifications.[26]

7.3.4 PRACTICAL CONSIDERATIONS

The clear message that this chapter has endeavoured to give is that the monitoring of glaucomatous visual field loss is severely hampered by variability. While the variability can be reduced by averaging the results from a large number of test locations, this approach runs the risk of failing to detect localised changes. An alternative approach is to use repeat measures of the visual field. The Normal Tension Glaucoma Study[27] is a good example of a repeat test strategy. In this study, any patient whose visual field changed by more than a small amount was subjected to a second confirmatory test within 1–4 weeks. However, the patient was not classified as progressing until a progressive change (initial and confirmatory test) was documented again 3 months later (i.e. progression was defined on the basis of four visual field examinations). The use of multistage criteria such as these obviously places a considerable extra burden upon heath service resources and it is in part for this reason that considerable effort has recently gone into developing new test strategies which retain the accuracy of the full threshold test while reducing the overall test time.[28]

Normally the ability of a visual field instrument to detect the presence of a visual field defect is subject to less variability than its ability to detect a change in the defect, because of the increased variability seen in the visual field once damage has occurred. In the normal eye the FOS curve is steep and the results repeatable. This consistency of responses has practical value when consideration is given to the fact that during the early stages of POAG visual field loss is normally confined to either the superior or inferior hemifield.

Practical advice

In the case of a patient whose visual field loss is confined to the superior hemifield the occurrence of a visual field defect in the inferior hemifield is clear evidence of progression. Ironically, when global measures of change are used this type of occurrence can easily be swamped by the noise in the damaged hemifield.

7.4 FINAL COMMENTS

This chapter has highlighted the many problems associated with the detection and monitoring of the visual field and the attempts that have been made to overcome these problems. No one would suggest that an ideal solution to the problems has been found but we think the reader of this chapter can appreciate that over the past few years our understanding of the problem has been enhanced and the direction of future research better defined. Before leaving the subject, it is important to reiterate that visual fields are a measure of visual function, the retention of which is the main objective of treatment. While disc and IOP measures might indicate that functional damage will occur or has already occurred, they are not, in themselves, a measure of that damage.

It is also important to emphasise that the treated rate of visual field loss can be very slow. Katz et al[29] reported that only 18% of eyes had >1 dB/year deterioration in the index *mean deviation* when followed up for 6 years. Detecting slow rates of change is always going to be difficult and involve long and expensive research programmes.

References

1. Armaly MF. Visual field defects in early open-angle glaucoma. Trans Am Ophthalmol Soc 1971; 69:147–162.

2. Henson DB, Artes PH, Chauhan BC. Diffuse loss of sensitivity in early glaucoma. Invest Ophthalmol Vis Sci 1999; 40:3147–3151.

3. Heijl A, Bengtsson B. Early visual field defects in glaucoma: A study of eyes developing field loss. In Bucci MG, ed. Glaucoma: Decision making in therapy. Berlin: Springer;1996.

4. Heijl A, Lindgren G, Lindgren A, et al. Extended empirical package for evaluation of single and multiple fields in glaucoma: STATPAC 2. In: Mills RP, Heijl A, eds. Perimetry Update 1990/1. Amsterdam: Kugler & Ghendini; 1991: 303–315.

5. Advanced glaucoma intervention study 2. Visual field test scoring and reliability. Ophthalmology 1994; 101:1445–1455.

6. Henson DB, Bryson H. Clinical results with the Henson-Hamblin CFS2000. Doc Ophthalmol Proc Series 1986; 49:233–238.

7. Hitchings RA. Outcome measures for glaucoma treatment. Br J Ophthalmol 1997; 81:427–428.

8. Werner EB, Drance SM. Early visual field disturbances in glaucoma. Arch Ophthalmol 1977; 95:1173–1175.

9. Henson DB, Chaudry S, Artes PH, et al. Response variability in the visual field: comparison of optic neuritis, glaucoma, ocular hypertension, and normal eyes. Invest Ophthalmol Vis Sci 2000; 41:417–421.

10. Weber J, Rau S. The properties of perimetric thresholds in normal and glaucomatous eyes. German J Ophthalmol 1992; 1:79–85.

11. Werner EB, Bishop KI, Koelle J, et al. A comparison of experienced clinical observers and statistical tests in detection of progressive field loss in glaucoma using automated perimetry. Acta Ophthalmol 1988; 106:619–623.

12. Hills JF, Johnson CA. Evaluation of the t test as a method of detecting visual field changes. Ophthalmology 1988; 95:261–266.

13. Holmin C, Krakau CET. Regression analysis of the central visual field in chronic glaucoma cases. Acta Ophthalmol 1982; 60:267 274.

14. O'Brien C, Schwartz B. The visual field in chronic open angle glaucoma: the rate of change in different regions of the field. Eye 1990; 4:557–562.

15. Noureddin BN, Poinoosawmy D, Fitzke FW, et al. Regression analysis of visual field progression in low tension glaucoma. Br J Ophthalmol 1991; 75:493–495.

16. Wild JM, Hussey MK, Flanagan JG, et al. Pointwise topographical and longitudinal modeling of the visual field in glaucoma. Invest Ophthalmol Vis Sci 1993; 34:1907–1916.

17. Fitzke FW, Hitchings RA, Poinoosawmy D, et al. Analysis of visual field progression in glaucoma. Br J Ophthalmol 1996; 80:40–48.

18. Viswanathan AC, Fitzke FW, Hitchings RA. Early detection of visual field progression in glaucoma: a comparison of PROGESSOR and STATPAC 2. Br J Ophthalmol 1997; 81.1037–1042.

19. Spencer IC, Spry PGD, Gray SF, et al. The Bristol shared care glaucoma study: study design. Ophthal Physiol Opt 1995; 15:391–394.

20. Henson DB, Spry PG, Spencer IC, et al. Variability in glaucomatous visual fields: implications for shared care schemes. Ophthal Physiol Opt 1998; 18.120–125.

21. Aulhorn E, Harms H. Early visual field defects in glaucoma. In: Leydhecker W, ed. Glaucoma. Tutzig Symposium, 1966. Basel: Karger; 1967: 151–175.

22. Drance SM. The early visual field defects in glaucoma. Invest Ophthalmol Vis Sci 1969; 9:84–91.

23. Hart WM, Becker B. The onset and evolution of glaucomatous visual field defects. Ophthalmology 1982; 89:268–279.

24. Jay JL, Murdoch JR. The rate of visual field loss in untreated primary open angle glaucoma. Br J Ophthalmol 1993; 77:176–178.

25. Henson DB, Spenceley S, Bull DR. Spatial classification of glaucomatous visual field loss. Brit J Ophthalmol 1996; 80:526–531.

26. Henson DB, Spenceley SE, Bull DR. Artificial neural network analysis of noisy visual field data in glaucoma. Artif Intell Med 1997; 10:99–113.

27. Schultzer M. Errors in the diagnosis of visual field progression in normal-tension glaucoma. Ophthalmology 1994; 101:1589–1595.

28. Bengtsson B, Olsson J, Heijl A, et al. A new generation of algorithms for computerised threshold perimetry, SITA. Acta Ophthalmol 1997; 75:368–375.

29. Katz J, Gilbert D, Quigley HA, et al. Estimating progression of visual field loss in glaucoma. Ophthalmology 1997; 104:1017–1025.

Chapter **8**

Diagnosis of the glaucomas 2: intraocular pressure

Robert Harper and David B Henson

CHAPTER CONTENTS

8.1 INTRODUCTION

The association between raised intraocular pressure (IOP) and glaucoma became established during the nineteenth century, although the role of IOP in causing glaucomatous visual field loss has since been the subject of much debate. Although raised IOP is accepted to be an important risk factor for the development of primary open angle glaucoma (POAG), the introduction of the concepts of 'normal tension glaucoma' (NTG) and 'ocular hypertension' (OHT) challenged the belief that a raised IOP was necessary for the development of POAG and that a raised IOP would always lead to the development of POAG. There has, therefore, been a change in perspective on the relation between IOP and POAG, with some definitions of POAG (e.g. Sponsel 1989[1] and Quigley 1993[2]) no longer considering elevated IOP as part of the definition of the disease.

While there is an increasing body of evidence linking glaucoma to vascular dysregulation,[3,4] there is also an accumulating body of evidence, from randomised trials, that reducing IOP exerts a favourable influence on the course of the disease. The trials include the Ocular Hypertension Treatment Study (OHTS), the Early Manifest Glaucoma Trial, the Advanced Glaucoma Intervention Study (AGIS), the Collaborative Normal Tension Glaucoma Study, and the Collaborative Initial Glaucoma Treatment Study. For a review of the main findings from these trials the reader is referred to the European Glaucoma Society.[5]

Collectively these trials show that IOP reduction is of benefit in OHT and glaucoma, and they also show that IOP lowering does not inevitably arrest the development of the disease.

In recent years there has also been increasing recognition of the importance of a number of factors, in particular corneal characteristics, in obtaining reliable estimates of IOP. Consequently, this change in perspective on IOP and glaucoma has been accompanied by a renewed interest in tonometry and the accuracy of our estimates of IOP. This chapter discusses:

- Definition of 'normal' IOP
- Factors which influence IOP
- Relationship of IOP to POAG
- Techniques of measurement of IOP and developments in tonometry
- Guidelines on referral.

The measurement of IOP is, of course, central to the management of those patients with established disease or those at risk of developing glaucoma, but it is beyond the scope of this chapter to discuss the control of IOP in these patients.

8.2 WHAT IS 'NORMAL' INTRAOCULAR PRESSURE?

Within the context of the disease process, 'normal' IOP could be considered to be the level at which no glaucomatous damage occurs; however, because individual susceptibility to optic nerve head damage will vary at a particular level of IOP, such a definition of 'normal' has little validity. 'Normal' IOP is usually, therefore, considered in relation to the distribution of IOP in the general population. Studies in non-glaucomatous populations show that the distribution of IOP is not Gaussian, but is positively skewed (i.e. towards higher levels of IOP). Figure 8.1 shows theoretical distributions of IOP in non-glaucomatous and glaucomatous populations. Epidemiological studies estimate the mean IOP in 'normal' eyes to be ~15–16 mmHg, with a standard deviation of ~2.5 mmHg. Although Gaussian statistics do not strictly apply, because of the skewed distribution, the upper limit of 'normal' is typically given as 21 mmHg (a figure which is approximately the

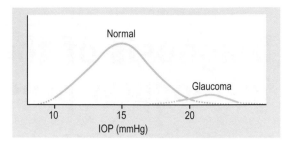

Fig. 8.1 Theoretical distributions of IOP in a non-glaucomatous and glaucomatous population. Note the considerable overlap in IOP values which occurs between these populations (Redrawn after Shields[6]).

mean IOP plus two standard deviations). When 'normal' IOP is referred to in this chapter, the meaning conveyed is that IOP is 21 mmHg or below. Whereas it would be convenient if this value, based on the statistical distribution of IOP, could be used as a simple cut-off criterion in screening for cases of POAG, the subsequent sections will demonstrate to readers that, unfortunately, such a strategy would not provide effective discrimination.

8.3 FACTORS INFLUENCING INTRAOCULAR PRESSURE

As discussed in Chapter 2, the level of IOP is determined by the rate of aqueous secretion, the resistance encountered in the outflow channels and the episcleral venous pressure. IOP tends to be higher in those individuals at risk for POAG. The IOP is, however, not constant in an individual and is subject to a number of influences that occur in the short term, in addition to the demographic, clinical and other factors that influence IOP in the longer term.

8.3.1 FACTORS CAUSING SHORT-TERM FLUCTUATIONS IN IOP

Arterial pulse

The arterial pulse creates a 2–3 mmHg oscillation in IOP known as the 'ocular pulse', i.e. the cyclic variation in IOP associated with the heartbeat.

Time of day (diurnal variation)

There is a tendency for IOP to be higher in the morning and lower in the afternoon and evening, although some studies have revealed peak IOP in the afternoon. There is some evidence to suggest that the characteristic mid-to-late afternoon depression in IOP is more significant in males.[7]

- The diurnal variation is typically ≤5 mmHg in 'normal' eyes, but is higher in ocular hypertensive or glaucomatous eyes.
- A diurnal variation of >10 mmHg is usually considered to be pathological.

The cause of this variation is unclear, although it might relate to the diurnal variation of plasma cortisol. Within the context of clinical practice where IOPs are recorded at a single point in time—the patient's appointment time—a large diurnal variation may lead to a failure to recognise a clinically abnormal IOP. There are no easy solutions to this problem.

Practical advice

- Within a screening context, it is recommended that those patients with *borderline* IOP should have repeat tonometry at an alternative time of day (preferably in the morning) to better inform the clinical decision.
- In theory, because in the majority of patients the IOP peak is in the morning, adopting a screening strategy which involved carrying out all tonometry early in the morning, especially in males, would reduce the number of false negatives; however, the feasibility of such a policy for population glaucoma screening or case finding would be problematic.
- For diagnosis, phasing (where IOP is monitored at different times during the course of the day, usually within the hospital) and home tonometry (where patients or their relatives may measure the IOP at different times of the day at home) are considered to be important tools in the assessment of some 'at-risk' patients, and to assess the level of IOP control in previously diagnosed and treated patients (e.g. patients with progressive field loss or optic disc changes in the presence of apparently 'normal' or 'controlled' IOP).

Contraction of intraocular and extraocular muscles

Contraction of both extraocular and intraocular muscles can increase IOP, for example, gaze away from the primary position or accommodation, although sustained accommodation can increase the outflow facility and produce a lowering of IOP. Blinking and, in particular, hard lid squeezing, have also been shown to increase IOP, although repeated lid squeezing can lead to a slight reduction in IOP.

Blood pressure, exertion and posture

IOP is known to increase by between 0.3 mmHg and 6 mmHg in both 'normal' and glaucomatous eyes when a subject changes from a sitting to a supine position. Although the magnitude of this postural influence is variable, it is known to be greater in glaucomatous eyes. An inverted position is even more likely to increase the IOP, probably due to elevated episcleral venous pressure, with the extent of the rise in IOP being related to the degree of inversion.

Depending on the nature of the activity, exertion can lead to either an increase or a decrease in IOP. For example, both short-term and prolonged aerobic exercise have been shown to lower IOP, with decreases of the order of ~25% being found in 'normal' individuals and ~30% being found in patients with glaucoma. In contrast, straining can increase IOP. For example, an increase due to raised episcleral venous pressure associated with Valsalva's manoeuvre (where there is forcible exhalation against the closed glottis, increasing intrathoracic pressure and impeding venous return to the heart). A tight collar or tie can increase IOP by up to 4 mmHg.[8] Similarly, holding one's breath can also cause a significant short-term elevation in IOP.

Fluid intake

Alcohol has been shown to lower IOP and caffeine to cause a small, transient increase in IOP, although it is unlikely that ordinary consumption of coffee causes a significant, sustained rise. Drinking a large quantity of water (~1 litre) generally increases IOP. The mechanism for the increase in IOP following water drinking is uncertain. The 'provocative' water drinking test, which was developed under the premise that the rise in IOP is greater in glaucomatous eyes, has been used to indirectly assess the facility of outflow, although the test is widely regarded to have limited diagnostic value.

Practical advice

All of the above factors are most likely to have a relatively short-term effect on the IOP. An awareness of these factors can alert optometrists about possible confounding factors, which in turn will assist in making clinical decisions about individual patients. If there is concern that any of these factors may have influenced IOP, repeat readings should be taken.

8.3.2 DEMOGRAPHIC, CLINICAL AND OTHER FACTORS INFLUENCING IOP

Age

In general, IOP is lower in young children and tends to rise with advancing age. The distribution of IOP has been found to be relatively Gaussian between the ages of 20 and 40 years, with the shift towards higher IOP with increasing age. A rise of between 1 mmHg and 2 mmHg has been found between the third and seventh decades of life. It is not clear whether this shift is due to a direct correlation between age and IOP or whether other factors such as blood pressure might account for the apparent association.

Sex

In the older age groups women have marginally higher IOP (~1–2 mmHg) than men, although the prevalence of glaucomatous damage is not greater in women.

Inheritance

The level of IOP in the general population appears to be genetically determined. Individuals with a first-degree relative with POAG and those with an enlarged C/D ratio tend to have higher IOP.

Race

Higher IOP has been reported in the non-glaucomatous black population. A higher mean IOP has also been reported in people born in Africa or Asia compared with those born in America or Europe.

Myopia

Several studies have found an association between myopia and raised IOP, although it is difficult to tease apart this association from the known relation between myopia and POAG.

Corneal characteristics

It has been recognised for many years that the properties of the cornea, including corneal thickness and curvature, elasticity and hydration, all influence the estimates of IOP obtained from tonometry. For example, an IOP reading higher than the true IOP will be recorded in an individual with a thicker than average cornea, whereas an IOP lower than the true IOP will be recorded in an individual with a thinner than average cornea. Similarly, a steeper than average cornea offers greater resistance to flattening in comparison with a flatter than average cornea, resulting in a relative over-estimation or underestimation of the true IOP, respectively (~1 mmHg/3D). In relation to corneal thickness, pachymetry is now regarded as an important adjunct to the assessment of ocular hypertension and glaucoma, not only so that estimates of IOP can be corrected for central corneal thickness,[9] but also because it is recognised from the OHTS that a knowledge of central corneal thickness provides important information about an individual's risk of developing glaucoma.[10] Unfortunately, no single correction factor is universally agreed upon, although clinically an error range of ~0.2–0.7 mmHg/10 μm difference from

Table 8.1 **Proportion of primary open angle glaucoma (POAG) with 'normal' intraocular pressure (IOP) 'at survey' for several large epidemiological studies**

Study location (author(s))	No. with POAG	Percentage with 'normal' IOP
Des Moines, USA (Armaly[11])	189	68
Ferndale, Wales (Hollows and Graham[12])	20	35
Framingham, USA (Leibowitz et al[13])	40	52
Baltimore, USA (Sommer et al[14])	194	59
Beaver Dam, USA (Klein et al[15])	104	32
Roscommon, Ireland (Coffey et al[16])	41	37
Blue Mountains, Australia (Mitchell et al[17])	108	75

an average central corneal thickness has been suggested.[5] Alternative forms of tonometry (see below) that might obviate the requirement to carry out pachymetry are currently being developed and marketed, although it may take several more years of research to determine the increased value of such instrumentation.

Systemic disease

There is evidence of an association between systemic hypertension and raised IOP, although the importance of this association in the development of POAG is not clear. An association between diabetes mellitus and raised IOP has also been found in a number of studies.

Ocular disease

In addition to the different ocular diseases which can increase IOP and cause secondary glaucoma, some ocular diseases actually reduce IOP. For example, acute anterior uveitis can cause a reduction in IOP (occasionally reducing the IOP to well below 10 mmHg) due to a decrease in the production of aqueous humour, and rhegmatogenous retinal detachments can cause a reduction in IOP due to reduced aqueous flow.

8.4 INTRAOCULAR PRESSURE AND POAG

Raised IOP is considered to be the most significant risk factor for POAG. Despite the fact that most epidemiological studies have found between one-third and two-thirds of all cases of POAG to have 'normal' IOP *at presentation* (see Table 8.1), the probability of glaucomatous optic nerve damage increases exponentially with higher pressures. The 'dose–response' relation between IOP and POAG provides supporting evidence for the role of IOP as a risk factor for POAG.

Many studies have examined the rate of conversion to glaucoma in OHT, and typically these studies have observed an incidence of visual field loss in approximately 1% of patients per year, although the wide variation in findings suggests that there are different degrees of susceptibility in the population with OHT. In the OHTS, the majority of cases of conversion to glaucoma were based upon the endpoint of optic nerve head change, and ~10% of subjects with OHT converted during the course of this 5-year study (i.e. ~90% of subjects with OHT did not convert). Although the conversion rate from OHT to glaucoma is relatively low, several studies have demonstrated that the higher the IOP, the greater the risk of developing POAG. For example:

- Leske[18] has shown that the overall risk of glaucomatous field loss is five times higher in people with IOP >21 mmHg than in people with lower IOP.
- Sommer et al[14] estimated in a multiracial population that those with IOP between 22 mmHg and 29 mmHg were 12.8 times more likely to develop POAG than people with IOP below 22 mmHg and those with IOP >30 mmHg

were 39 times more likely to develop POAG.

Also, research has demonstrated a relation between raised IOP and the extent of visual field loss at presentation. However, some research needs to be interpreted with caution because of the possibility of 'work-up bias' (i.e. before inclusion, subjects had to satisfy certain criteria in respect to their IOP and visual fields, which meant they may not have been a truly random sample). In treated glaucoma cases, the relation between the IOP and the progression of visual field loss has been more difficult to establish, although AGIS indicates that a dose–response relation between IOP and visual field progression is likely. AGIS findings suggest that eyes with an IOP <18 mmHg at all visits over a 6-year period will not show progression of their initial visual field defect, whereas eyes with worse control (i.e. some follow-up visits with an IOP >18 mmHg) are more likely to show progression.

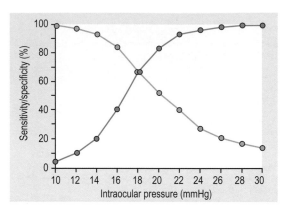

Fig. 8.2 Sensitivity and specificity curves for IOP as a screening test for glaucoma (drawn from the data of the Baltimore Eye Survey[19]). The curves illustrate the trade-off in test sensitivity and test specificity as the criterion for classifying a subject as glaucomatous/ non-glaucomatous is systematically varied. Note that no single cut-off criterion has both high sensitivity and high specificity.

8.5 SENSITIVITY AND SPECIFICITY OF TONOMETRY FOR DETECTING POAG

A number of studies have evaluated the effectiveness of glaucoma screening tests, including tonometry. Probably the most representative data is from the population-based Baltimore Eye Study.[19] The data indicate that no single IOP cut-off criterion has both high sensitivity and high specificity (Fig. 8.2). The relatively high percentage of patients with POAG having IOP within the 'normal' range at the time of presentation was noted above (see section 8.3), and it should come as no surprise to learn from Fig. 8.2 that an IOP cut-off criterion of >21 mmHg has limited sensitivity (detection rate) (~50%).

Practical advice

The sensitivity/specificity curves, illustrated in Fig. 8.2, show that tonometry is an ineffective detection test when used in isolation. Reasonable levels of sensitivity and specificity for effective detection of POAG are best achieved by employing the combination of tonometry, visual field assessment and optic disc evaluation.[20]

8.6 PREDICTIVE POWER OF TONOMETRY

In making clinical decisions on the basis of tonometric readings, it is important to know the likelihood or probability of having POAG at each level of IOP. One approach to deriving probability estimates for the likelihood of POAG is to consider the actual number of 'normal' and glaucomatous eyes in a population over a wide range of IOP values. This approach has been previously used by Davanger et al[21] in a large population-based study of older Norwegians. Their data (Fig. 8.3) show that:

- At an IOP of ~18 mm Hg, the probability of having POAG is near zero.
- At ~28 mm Hg, the probability is 0.6.
- At ~35 mm Hg, the probability approaches 1.0 (i.e. approaches certainty).

It is important to remember that the low probability of POAG at 'normal' levels of IOP is a reflection of the prevalence of POAG in the general population. Indeed, these probability estimates are quite consistent with a significant percentage of all POAG cases having IOP within the

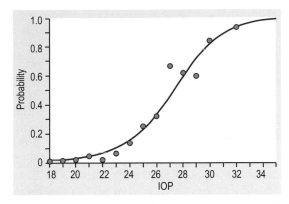

Fig. 8.3 Empirically derived probability curve showing the likelihood of glaucoma for a range of intraocular pressure values (redrawn from the data of Davanger et al, 1991[21]).

'normal' range (as the epidemiological data suggest), but given the very large number of 'normal' individuals with IOP within the same range, the probability estimates for POAG are correspondingly low.

Practical advice

- Within the context of POAG detection, arguably tonometry in isolation provides useful information (i.e. a reduction of uncertainty in the clinical decision) only when the IOP is raised outside the 'normal' range, and that it is even more important to use other detection tests when the recorded IOP is 'normal'. Although this latter approach to sequential clinical testing may appear to be counterintuitive, superficially at least, it actually represents a more rational approach to decision making.
- Another approach to deriving probability estimates is to use Bayesian statistics or likelihood ratios. Given a test result, a likelihood ratio measures how many times more likely a subject with disease is to have that test result than a subject without the disease.[22]

8.7 MEASUREMENT OF INTRAOCULAR PRESSURE: TONOMETRY

While IOP can be experimentally measured directly by cannulation, in clinical practice IOP is estimated by tonometry. Tonometers can be classified in simple terms into those that indent the cornea and those that applanate the cornea, although some instruments, including the Tonopen, are more difficult to classify. Indentation tonometry is largely of historical interest, and will not be considered further here.

8.7.1 APPLANATION TONOMETRY

Applanation tonometry is based upon the Imbert–Fick law, which, when applied to the eye, states that the IOP is equal to the weight applied to the cornea (in g) divided by the applanated area (in mm^2). Strictly speaking, this law is correct only for a spherical container with an infinitely thin, flexible, elastic and dry limiting membrane (i.e. a container which would create no resistance to flattening and allow expansion elsewhere so that the container pressure would not increase/decrease with applanation). The two most widely used applanation tonometers are the Goldmann contact applanation tonometer and non-contact tonometers (NCTs).

Goldmann applanation tonometry

The Goldmann tonometer measures the force required to applanate a circular area of 3.06 mm diameter. This diameter was chosen for three reasons:

1. The amount of fluid displaced with such a small applanated area is minimal, thus, although the walls of the eye have some rigidity, the IOP at measurement is almost identical to the true IOP.
2. Goldmann's studies showed that for applanated areas of 3–4 mm diameter, the surface tension force from the corneal film, which tends to pull the tonometer cone towards the eye, is equal but opposite to the force of corneal resistance. As a result the tonometer force is equal to the IOP.

3. When a diameter of 3.06 mm is used, the conversion between tonometer force and IOP is simple, i.e. force (in g) × 10 = IOP (in mmHg).

The Goldmann tonometer, because it has been the instrument of choice for many years, is not only widely regarded as the best measurement tool for clinical decision making in glaucoma, but it has also become the 'gold standard' or validating criterion against which all other tonometers are compared. The accuracy of the Goldmann tonometer in manometric studies is good, although early work by Moses and Liu[23] found that repeated measures with the Goldmann differed by 2 mmHg or more in 35% of cases. A subsequent early study on repeat readings by Thorburn[24] found good intraobserver test-retest repeatability (the standard deviation of differences was <1 mmHg) although, as one might expect, poorer interobserver repeatability (the standard deviation of differences was ~1.6 mmHg). Slightly lower reliability might be expected for the hand-held version of the Goldmann (Perkins tonometer).

In addition to these advantages, the instrument has a simple robust design which also helps to make it the instrument of choice within ophthalmology and optometric co-management. Despite the advantages, however, errors can arise in Goldmann tonometry, in addition to those considered in section 8.3.2 (Corneal characteristics), and these include the following:

- The width of the tears' meniscus may influence the IOP readings, with wider menisci causing slightly higher estimates. Ideally, the width of the semicircles should be about one-tenth of the diameter applanated (i.e. ~0.3 mm, although they will appear to be ~3 mm with 10× magnification).
- Incorrect vertical alignment of the semicircles can also result in a higher reading, because vertical decentration of the prism will require a larger force to match the inner edges of the 'semicircles'.
- If the eyelids touch the probe an increased IOP can be recorded, producing an effect similar to that caused by blinking/lid squeezing.
- Prolonged contact between the cone and the cornea can cause an apparent decrease in IOP (in addition to potential corneal damage) due to

the effect of 'aqueous massage'. Over a five minute period, the IOP can gradually fall by ~3–4 mmHg on repeated readings.

- If liquids other than water are used to wet the fluorets, the surface tension of the tears can be altered (minimal effect only). Similarly, if liquids are used to clean the tonometer head, these should have appropriate wetting characteristics.
- If corneal astigmatism is greater than 3.00D then an elliptical area of corneal contact can occur. In cases of high astigmatism, the flattest meridian must be aligned at 43° to the apex of the cone. An irregular cornea will also distort the semicircles and interfere with the accuracy of the measured IOP.
- If the tonometer is not regularly calibrated, systematic or random errors can result.

As is the case with all tonometers which contact the eye, there is the risk of transmitting infection. Disinfection of the tonometer cone is, therefore, essential, although the introduction of disposable tips has removed this potential difficulty. In addition, there is the requirement to anaesthetise the cornea.

Non-contact tonometry

The first NCT was designed by Grolman[25] and introduced by American Optical in 1972, although the principle was considered as early as 1951 by Erich Zeiss. Currently at least eight different NCTs are commercially available (the Reichert (formerly American Optical) NCT II and auto NCT AT550 and portable PT100 instruments, the Keeler Pulsair EasyEye, the Topcon CT80/80A, the Nidek NT-2000/4000, the Kowa KT-500 and the Canon TX-10).

The original NCT directed an air-puff towards the cornea. The point of applanation by the air-puff was detected by an optical system, and the time taken from the onset of the puff to the applanation of the cornea was recorded electronically. This time is related to the IOP. In contrast, the later generations of NCT measure the air-pulse pressure within the instrument chamber at the moment of applanation. This measure has been found to correlate well with IOP, and is less sensitive to the effect of mechanical wear. In contrast with most instruments, the portable Keeler Pulsair is a hand-held instrument which can be used in any position and does not require the use of a chin rest for alignment. This instrument creates a ramped air pulse which automatically applanates the cornea at alignment. An optical system detects the applanation and initiates the sampling of the pulse pressure within the instrument. A revised and recalibrated version of the Keeler Pulsair (the '2000') was introduced in 1991 and the current fourth generation instrument is known as the Pulsair 'EasyEye'. The Topcon NCT was introduced in 1988 and has undergone several changes since. This instrument also samples the pulse pressure within the tonometer and converts it to an estimate of the IOP. In common with other modern NCTs, this instrument uses a lower pulse pressure than the original Reichert instrument. For an account of the design features of the early NCTs see Henson.[26]

In general, the principal advantages of NCT over contact tonometry include the following:

- The measurements can be made without the need for an anaesthetic.
- The risk of damage to the corneal surface is considerably reduced.
- The non-contact instruments are less sensitive to the effects of operator technique.
- The use of repeat measures is unlikely to change the IOP.
- There is an extremely small risk of infection or cross contamination.
- IOP can be recorded rapidly.
- Non-contact instruments are more acceptable for use in children or in individuals in whom tolerance to contact presents difficulties.
- Non-contact instruments can be used by trained non-clinically qualified staff, thus increasing the feasibility of more widespread screening.

It is of course fair to point out that some of these advantages could become limitations if the user of the NCT is unaware of the errors that can be introduced in estimating the IOP (e.g. the variations in IOP considered in section 8.2). For example, with all NCTs it is essential to take at least three to four readings per eye in order to balance out the effect of the ocular pulse (see section 8.3.1). With the Goldmann tonometer, a single measure is usually adequate because the ocular

pulse is visible at the point of applanation in the form of an oscillation of the semicircles, thus presenting the opportunity to record an average endpoint.

The findings of some of the method-comparison studies (which have examined the accuracy of non-contact tonometers in relation to the Goldmann instrument) have been reviewed. The vast majority of these studies conclude that NCTs provide clinically meaningful measures of IOP which equate to those obtained by the Goldmann instrument. Despite these studies, and the many advantages listed above, NCT has not replaced Goldmann tonometry as the technique of choice in the hospital setting.

Regression towards the mean effect

There is some evidence that the accuracy of NCTs is still doubted by many clinicians, a large proportion of whom believe, at least to some extent, that the instruments 'read high'.[27] This belief, which is counter to the results from published comparison studies, is probably due to a combination of factors. One of these is that method-comparison studies are likely to use highly trained people to take readings whereas in a clinical setting they are more likely to be used by staff with less training in tonometry. A second factor is the regression to the mean effect. Henson and Harper[27] have proposed that an explanation for the discrepancy between the published clinical evaluations of NCTs and the observations noted in ophthalmic departments could be the way in which optometrists select cases for referral, combined with the variability inherent in the measurement of IOP. While most optometrists use a combination of different tests, and not simply an IOP reading, when deciding whether or not to refer a patient with suspect glaucoma, they are occasionally presented with a situation where the measured IOP is high and the optic discs and visual fields appear normal (see example in Fig. 8.4). Under these circumstances, optometrists may use a simple cut-off criterion for referral (e.g. if the IOP is >28 mmHg, then refer). Because IOP is affected by a number of sources of variation, sometimes one will obtain extreme values just by chance; however, these readings will, on average, be lower when repeated, thus lying

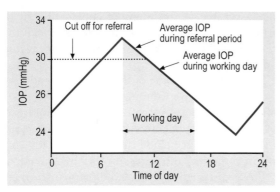

Fig. 8.4 Regression towards the mean example (after Henson and Harper[27]), using diurnal variation as the source of variability. The intraocular pressure (IOP) has been assumed to vary in a linear fashion with a single peak at 9.00 am for the purposes of making the calculations simple. If the patient is examined between the hours of 9.00 am and 11.00 am and the optometrist uses a 30 mmHg cut-off criterion for referral, then they will be referred. If the patient's appointment time within the hospital lies within the working day, the average IOP during this period will be 28 mmHg. Thus the patient's IOP will, on average, be lower than that specified in the optometrist's letter.

closer to the mean value of the true IOP than the first reading. The effect just described represents a sampling phenomenon, known as the 'regression towards the mean' effect[28] and is likely to occur regardless of the form of tonometry used in the primary care setting.

Practical advice

Although the sampling bias just described cannot be removed, the practice of repeating measures of IOP prior to referral and the recording of these findings in any subsequent referral is often helpful to the ophthalmologist, especially in patients in whom the level of IOP is considered to be the principal reason for referral.

8.7.2 DEVELOPMENTS IN TONOMETRY

Pneumotonometry gives a continuous measurement of IOP from which the magnitude of the

ocular pulse can be measured. The relationship between changes in blood volume and the ocular pulse at a known heart rate enables the pulsatile ocular blood flow to be estimated. Since a reduction in pulsatile ocular blood flow has been documented in patients with POAG and NTG, it is suggested that the non-invasive measurement of this pulsatile component of ocular blood flow might provide valuable information on the vascular aetiology of POAG.[29] While the pneumatic measurement of IOP has a long history, being first introduced in the 1960s by Langham, interest has been renewed following the development of the ocular blood flow (OBF) tonometer. The OBF tonometer comprises a compact base unit with data storage facility, a sensor (which attaches to a slit lamp) and a printer. This portable instrument automatically generates a measure of pulsatile ocular blood flow and it takes no longer than the measurement of IOP by the Goldmann tonometer. The instrument has been shown to provide reproducible measures;[29] however, a more recent study has questioned the value of the OBF pneumotonometer as a tool for measuring IOP,[30] and, contrary to expectations, based on the mechanism of measurement of IOP, corneal thickness appears to affect measures obtained with the OBF tonometer more than they affect Goldmann measures.[31]

The possible errors in IOP estimates introduced by variations in the properties of the cornea were discussed briefly in section 8.3.2. Manufacturers have been quick to try to deal with this limitation by facilitating the use of pachymetry in ophthalmic practice. Several different models that provide correction estimates for IOP measures are commercially available, including one instrument that combines tonometry and pachymetry within a single unit. Potentially of even greater interest is the development of the Reichert Ocular Response Analyser, currently undergoing clinical evaluation. This NCT-like instrument employs a dynamic bi-directional applanation process to provide a measure of 'corneal hysteresis'. It is suggested that this new parameter reveals the viscoelastic properties of the cornea and can determine the total corneal resistance (including the aggregate effects of thickness, rigidity and hydration) to the force of the tonometer during IOP estimation, although the results from clinical trials are necessary before informed comment can be made on the value of this type of measurement in managing patients. The same point might also be made for dynamic contour tonometry (DCT), a totally new method of measuring IOP based on the principle of contour matching. The DCT tip features a concave surface with a contact surface of 7 mm and a miniaturized piezoresistive sensor built flush with the centre of the contact surface. The Pascal DCT is slit lamp mounted and operated in a similar fashion to the Goldmann. IOP readings are sampled continuously and both IOP and ocular pulse amplitude data can be displayed. It is suggested that the DCT provides IOP readings that are not influenced by corneal thickness and one recent study suggests IOP values are closer to manometric levels with this instrument than IOP values recorded by the Goldmann.[32]

8.8 IOP REFERRAL GUIDELINES IN ROUTINE OPTOMETRIC PRACTICE

IOP is a major risk factor for POAG, and the higher the IOP, the greater the risk; however, referrals for an ophthalmological opinion must be made with knowledge of other test data and other risk factors. In view of the variability of IOP measures, it is better to repeat tests in equivocal cases, rather than make an immediate referral. Because of the diurnal variation of IOP, it is also helpful for future comparisons to record time of day on the record card and also in any referral note to an ophthalmologist. The nature of clinical opinion and the variations in local circumstances dictate that the following criteria are offered as guidelines only:

- For markedly raised IOP, refer when repeated measures of the IOP are >28–30 mmHg, even if the optic nerve head and visual field are normal.
- Consider the risk of a central retinal vein occlusion. An IOP >35 mmHg requires a semi-urgent referral.
- Consider the inter-eye difference in IOP. An inter-eye difference of ≤4 mmHg is regarded as 'normal', 5–7 mmHg is suspect and ≥8 mmHg is usually abnormal.

8.9 FINAL COMMENTS

This chapter has highlighted some of the limitations of tonometry; however, it is worth remembering that, historically, the lowering of IOP has been the only treatment option available to clinicians and that the achievement of a specific 'target' IOP was widely viewed as the final arbiter of the 'success' of glaucoma treatment. Despite the subsequent change in emphasis placed on the role of IOP in relation to the pathogenesis and management of glaucoma, the measurement of IOP will continue to be a major factor in the management of this disease in the foreseeable future. Results of a number of recent randomised trials provide a greater evidence base upon which to form management decisions in respect of both the risk of glaucoma development and the risk of glaucoma progression.

References

1. Sponsel WE. Tonometry in Question: Can visual screening tests play a more decisive role in glaucoma diagnosis and management? Surv Ophthalmol 1989; 33:291–300.
2. Quigley HA. Open angle glaucoma. New Engl J Med 1993; 328:1097–1105.
3. Hayreh SS. Factors influencing blood flow in the optic nerve head. J Glaucoma 1997; 6:412–425.
4. Cioffi GA. Three common assumptions about ocular blood flow and glaucoma. Surv Ophthalmol 2001; 45 Suppl 3:S325–S331; discussion S332–S334.
5. European Glaucoma Society. Terminology and guidelines for glaucoma, 2nd edn. European Glaucoma Society; 2003.
6. Shields MB. Textbook of Glaucoma, 4th edn. Baltimore: Williams & Wilkins; 1998.
7. Pointer JS. The diurnal variation of intraocular pressure in non-glaucomatous subjects: relevance in a clinical context. Ophthal Physiol Opt 1997; 17:456–465.
8. Teng C, Gurses-Ozden R, Liebmann JM, et al. Effect of a tight necktie on intraocular pressure. Br J Ophthalmol 2003; 87:946–948.

9. Doughty MJ, Zaman ML. Human corneal thickness and its impact on intraocular pressure measures: a review and meta-analysis approach. Surv Ophthalmol 2000; 44:367–408.

10. Brandt JD. Corneal thickness in glaucoma screening, diagnosis and management. Curr Opin Ophthalmol 2004; 15:85–89.

11. Armaly MF. On the distribution of applanation pressure and arcuate scotoma. In: Patterson G, Miller SJH, Patterson GD, eds. Drug Mechanisms in Glaucoma. London: Churchill Livingstone, 1996.

12. Hollows FC, Graham PA. Intraocular pressure, glaucoma and glaucoma suspects in a defined population. Br J Ophthalmol 1966; 50:570–586.

13. Leibowitz HM, Krueger DE, Maunder LR, et al. The Framingham Eye Study monograph: An ophthalmological and epidemiological study of cataract, glaucoma, diabetic retinopathy, macular degeneration, and visual acuity in a general population of 2631 adults, 1973–1975. Surv Ophthalmol 1980; 24 (Suppl):335–610.

14. Sommer A, Tielsch JM, Katz J, et al. Relationship between intraocular pressure and primary open angle glaucoma among white and black Americans. Arch Ophthalmol 1991; 109:1090–1095.

15. Klein BEK, Klein R, Sponsel WE, et al. Prevalence of glaucoma. The Beaver Dam Study. Ophthalmology 1992; 99:1499–1504.

16. Coffey M, Reidy A, Wormald R, et al. Prevalence of glaucoma in the west of Ireland. Br J Ophthalmol 1993; 77:17–21.

17. Mitchell P, Smith W, Attebo K, et al. Prevalence of open-angle glaucoma in Australia. The Blue Mountains Study. Ophthalmology 1996; 103:1661–1669.

18. Leske MC. The epidemiology of open angle glaucoma: a review. Am J Epidemiol 1983; 118:166–191.

19. Tielsch JM, Katz J, Singh K, et al. A population based evaluation of glaucoma screening: The Baltimore Eye Survey. Am J Epidemiol 1991; 134:1102–1110.

20. Harper R, Reeves B. Glaucoma Screening: the importance of combined test data. Optom Vis Sci 1999; 75: 537–543.

21. Davanger M, Ringvold A, Blika S. The probability of having glaucoma at different IOP levels. Acta Ophthalmol 1991; 69:565–568.

22. Harper R, Henson D, Reeves B. Appraising evaluations of screening/diagnostic tests: the importance of the study populations. Br J Ophthalmol 2000; 84:1198–1202.

23. Moses RA, Liu CH. Repeated applanation tonometry. Am J Ophthalmol 1968; 66:89.

24. Thorburn W. The accuracy of clinical applanation tonometry. Acta Ophthalmol 1978; 56:1.

25. Grolman B. A new tonometer system. Am J Optom Arch Am Acad Optom 1972; 49:646.

26. Henson DB. Tonometers. In: Optometric Instrumentation, 2nd edn. Oxford: Butterworth-Heinemann, 1996.

27. Henson DB, Harper RA. Do non-contact tonometers read high? Ophthalmic Physiol Opt 1998; 18:308–310.

28. Bland JM, Altman DG. Some examples of regression towards the mean. BMJ 1994; 309:780.

29. Butt Z, O'Brien C. Reproducibility of pulsatile ocular blood flow measurements. J Glaucoma 1995; 4:214–218.

30. Bhan A, Bhargava J, Vernon SA, et al. Repeatability of ocular blood flow pneumotonometry. Ophthalmology 2003; 110:1551–1554.

31. Gunvant P, Baskaran M, Vijaya L, et al. Effect of corneal parameters on measurements using the pulsatile ocular blood flow tonograph and Goldmann applanation tonometer. Br J Ophthalmol 2004; 88:518–522.

32. Kniestedt C, Nee M, Stamper R. Dynamic contour tonometry: A comparative study on human cadaver eyes. Arch Ophthalmol 2004; 122:1287–1293.

Chapter 9

Diagnosis of glaucoma through examination of the optic nerve head

Sarah J Wilson, Simon JA Rankin, Colm O'Brien and Yvonne Delaney

CHAPTER CONTENTS

9.1 INTRODUCTION

The optic nerve is the defining pathological feature of glaucoma. Most definitions of glaucoma would now be based on a description of an optic neuropathy that leads to characteristic visual field defects which may be associated with raised intraocular pressure. This optic neuropathy which causes a characteristic change in the optic nerve head known as cupping is and has been recognised for over a century as being specific to glaucoma. Initially it was thought that the optic disc was swollen in glaucoma, but then it was realised that the characteristic change was an excavation of the central region of the optic nerve head. Since then an elaborate science has been established based on the examination of the optic disc, the interpretation of the findings seen and their significance in potential glaucoma.

It is essential that practitioners screening for glaucoma have a good knowledge of the normal optic disc and its variation throughout the population.[1] They must also be skilled in its evaluation. Although the diagnosis of glaucoma depends on the inter-relationship of the triad—intraocular pressure, cupping of the optic disc and visual field defects—good screening is heavily dependent on accurate optic disc analysis. The significance of intraocular pressure and visual field testing are discussed in Chapters 1, 5, 7 and 8. However the difficulties in carrying out accurate

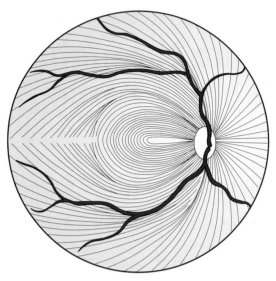

Fig. 9.1   This figure illustrates the retinal nerve fibre layer pattern. The papillomacular bundle travels straight from the macula to the disc. Temporal to the fovea, the bundles of axons make their way around this forming the typical arcuate pattern entering the superior or inferior poles of the optic disc. No axons cross the horizontal raphé.

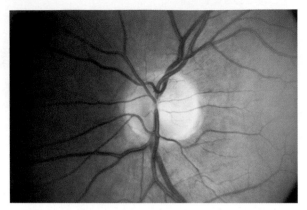

Fig. 9.2   A normal optic disc. There is a shallow central cup with a C/D ratio of approximately 0.3. The edge of the disc is poorly defined because of the thickness of the nerve fibre layer. The striations of the normal retinal nerve fibre layer can be seen converging on the disc.

automated threshold–related visual field screening techniques on older patients means that many false positives will be avoided by good disc analysis and early cases of glaucoma will be detected before potentially disabling visual field deterioration develops.

9.2 NORMAL ANATOMY AND PHYSIOLOGY

The optic nerve is composed of approximately one million axons which originate from cell bodies of the ganglion cell layer of the retina and ultimately synapse in the lateral geniculate body. The axons lie on the retina forming the characteristic pattern of the retinal nerve fibre layer (Fig. 9.1). As these bundles of axons approach the scleral canal they are organised so that those axons from more peripheral retinal sites are deepest within the retina turning at right angles and cascading over the rim while those axons from more central regions occupy a more superficial site on the retina and

cascade over the top of the deeper fibres so taking up a more central position on the optic disc.[2]

As these axons cascade into the scleral canal, they fill it to form the optic nerve head and ultimately the optic nerve. The scleral canal varies in size largely depending on the size of the globe overall. The size of the canal determines the size of the optic nerve head. As there appears to be a relatively constant number of axons in the normal retina and optic nerve head it means that they will occupy a similar area of the optic nerve head no matter what size the whole structure is. The area that they form is termed the neuroretinal rim and the space that is left in the centre of the optic disc is the cup. The size of the cup therefore varies with the overall size of the optic disc. This cup is an excavation in the optic nerve head above the level of the lamina cribrosa that lies at the level of the sclera and represents the wall of the globe.

The normal optic disc is shaped as a vertical ovoid. The cup sits within this centrally and may be round or a horizontal ovoid. It is displaced slightly superiorly so that the thickest area of neuroretinal rim is the inferior. This is because the fovea sits slightly below the horizontal centre of the optic disc and the papillomacular bundle arising from it with its huge density of nerve fibres adds extra bulk to the inferior portion of the optic disc. The rim is next thickest superiorly followed by the nasal and temporal rims. A normal optic disc is illustrated in Fig. 9.2.

The area of the optic disc varies between approximately $1.25\,mm^2$ and $4.5\,mm^2$. The mean area is $2.2 \pm 0.5\,mm^2$. Small discs are often typical of a hypermetropic eye which has a shorter axial length and more 'crowding' of the structures present. In comparison, large discs are often characteristic of myopic eyes with an increased axial length. The optic disc is approximately 12% larger in black people than in white people.[1]

The cup is measured by judging its vertical height against the vertical height of the optic disc. This is expressed as a ratio—the cup/disc ratio. In normal eyes the cup/disc ratio is generally below 0.5. There is usually symmetry between the two eyes and a discrepancy of >0.2 in the cup/disc ratio is uncommon in a normal situation. If there is asymmetry between the sizes of the optic disc in the two eyes, an asymmetry of the cup corresponding to the respective disc sizes would be expected. This asymmetry would often be predictable from the refractive status of the two eyes. Approximately 10% of people have a cup/disc ratio greater than 0.5.[3]

The neuroretinal rim should be considered more important than the cup. It represents neural tissue that is present rather than the cup, which is negative space. The neural rim is like a doughnut surrounding the cup and particularly in smaller discs should have a convexity into the vitreous due to the density of nerve fibres composing it. The blood vessels, the central retinal artery and vein, show great variation in their pathways out of this region. In general they arise nasally in the cup and slant nasally onto that wall of the cup before branching and ascending the superior or inferior cup walls and passing over or through the neural rim tissue. Cilioretinal arteries occur in approximately 25% of people and most often arise from the temporal rim of the disc. They are so called as they arise from the short posterior ciliary arteries that are supplying the choroid and deeper regions of the optic nerve head. The circumlinear vessel arises from the central retinal artery and curves around the upper or lower border of the cup before proceeding onto the retina.

9.3 EXAMINATION AND EVALUATION

The direct ophthalmoscope has been the most popular instrument used in examination of the disc. It allows a relatively easy approach to examining the disc for both patient and practitioner. Although dilation of the pupil is helpful for improving the view available, with modern instruments with halogen co-axial optics, the technique provides the most accessible view of the disc through an undilated pupil. The view obtained is an upright and magnified monocular image. The whole disc can usually be seen within one field of the beam and this helps in the assessment of the size of the optic disc. The specifications of different manufacturers vary. Using the 5° aperture of the Welch–Allyn direct ophthalmoscope a beam of light is projected onto the retina with a diameter of approximately $1.5\,mm$ and an area of $1.77\,mm^2$. If this beam is placed on the retina adjacent to the optic disc a comparative estimation of size can be made. The normal optic disc with an area of approximately $2.2\,mm^2$ should be 15% larger than the beam's area. Experienced practitioners show a good ability to judge the optic disc size using this method. The beam should sit just inside the margins of a normally sized optic disc. The major part of the examination is carried out with a white light, but the red-free light can be used to examine vascular details such as a disc haemorrhage and also the retinal nerve fibre layer as it approaches the disc.

Clinicians have increasingly used the slit lamp in conjunction with high-powered convex lenses to examine the disc (Fig. 9.3). These range in their strength, the most suitable being the +90D, +78D and +66D lenses. Each of these conveys slightly differing views. The 66D gives the greatest magnification whereas the 90D allows limited examination through an undilated pupil. These lenses, in general, require pupillary dilation to achieve a view of the disc. The lens is hand-held approximately 1 cm in front of the eye while the co-axial slit lamp is retreated until a focused view is obtained. The view is inverted and magnified and, most importantly, through a dilated pupil it is binocular, allowing stereoscopic assessment. As the disc and the cup are three-dimensional structures this confers

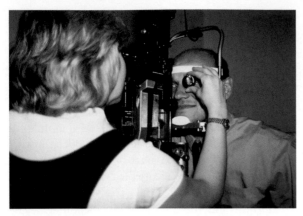

Fig. 9.3 A patient being examined with a convex +66D lens at the slit lamp allowing a binocular and stereoscopic view.

great advantage and many would regard this as the most accurate method of disc assessment. The stereoscopic view does tend to give an impression of a larger cup than when viewed with a direct ophthalmoscope. These lenses can also be used to measure the vertical height of the optic disc using the micrometer scale of a Haag-Streit slit lamp allowing an estimate of the overall size of the disc.[4] Using the 90D Volk indirect aspheric lens and the Haag-Streit slit lamp the range of normal values obtained in the emmetropic eye (±3D) is from 1.2 mm to 1.6 mm with a mean of 1.4 mm. These values are specific for the Volk lens and the Haag-Streit slit lamp. Therefore any disc which has a vertical height of 1.6 mm or greater is a large optic disc whereas measurements of 1.2 mm or less represent a small optic disc. This is an accurate and reliable method to measure optic disc size.

Using the slit lamp, a contact lens such as a Goldmann 3-mirror lens can also be used. While this provides a stereoscopic upright and magnified view of the disc the necessity to use a contact technique with a viscous tear preparation to maintain a meniscus between the lens and the cornea is a significant disadvantage. The Hruby lens, a −55D lens, is still fitted to many slit lamps and allows disc examination. It is difficult to use and provides a small field of view.

Finally, the examiner must find the best method to document what has been seen to allow the original or a subsequent examiner to detect a change in these features at any subsequent examination. The first stage of documentation would be the cup/disc ratio. As the different methods of examination may produce a discrepancy in the apparent cup/disc ratio, a note should be made of which method was used to view the disc. Simple descriptive phrases can then be added to this. A drawing can be made giving an impression of the shape and size of the cup and specific features such as a haemorrhage. Each of these methods is an improvement on the previous but it must be realised that they have all been shown to be extremely prone to misjudgements of reproducibility. This means that sequential judgement of change over a long period of time may be difficult. For this reason most glaucoma services would now consider imaging the optic disc at least at presentation so that any change in the future can be judged in comparison to this. Although simple comments may suffice in a screening environment prior to possible referral of a suspicious disc, it is not sufficient to rely on a cup measurement or a line drawing in a situation of co-management. Photographic documentation is relatively inexpensive. Other techniques such as scanning laser ophthalmoscopes remain expensive and require experienced technical staff to manage them. This makes them likely to be accessible only to central glaucoma units and their images can be distributed to more distant clinical users by document or digital transfer.

These techniques, which are described later in the chapter, provide the method of examination but the evaluation of what is seen is the art of glaucoma screening. The examiner must use a combination of these techniques to be able to build a three-dimensional perspective of the optic disc and its size. This is then central to the decision-making processes in the management of the patient.

9.4 FEATURES OF THE OPTIC DISC

9.4.1 CUP/DISC RATIO

The major feature of the disc in the evaluation of possible glaucoma is the cupping of the disc. The features of a normal cup have been described. The cup is an excavation and is surrounded by walls ascending to the neural rim and retina. To assess the cup an evaluation must be made as to what

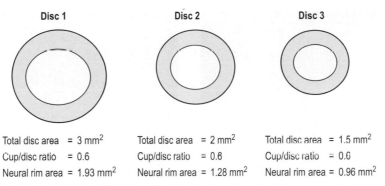

Disc 1

Disc 2

Disc 3

Total disc area = 3 mm^2	Total disc area = 2 mm^2	Total disc area = 1.5 mm^2
Cup/disc ratio = 0.6	Cup/disc ratio = 0.6	Cup/disc ratio = 0.6
Neural rim area = 1.93 mm^2	Neural rim area = 1.28 mm^2	Neural rim area = 0.96 mm^2

Fig. 9.4   A scale drawing of three optic discs of different physiological sizes. Each disc has a cup/disc ratio of 0.6. Despite the initial impression based on the absolute size of the cup, the neural rim area is in fact the measurement that denotes how much functional tissue is present. In disc 1 the neural rim area is huge and normal, in disc 2 the neural rim area is reasonable and may be pathological or physiological. In disc 3 the neural rim area is small and almost certainly implies pathological erosion.

constitutes the edge of the cup or the contour. In a deep cup with steep sides this is rather easy as the edge of the cup may appear as a sharp 90° corner. However if the cup is rather less deep and more poorly defined the cup is not as definitively outlined and is much more difficult to measure with certainty. The cup rim usually coincides with the level of the retina, the healthy doughnut shaped neural rim may lie slightly above it. The rim is most clearly delineated in the nasal portion which is relatively steep and has the central retinal vessels positioned against it. The superior and inferior rims would be the next most prominent, often with a well-defined neural edge and with vessels turning over the edge to advance onto the retina (bayoneting). The temporal edge of the cup is generally the most difficult to define as it constitutes a sloping surface from the angle that the optic nerve inserts into the globe with the axons ascending the slope to form the papillomacular bundle on the retina. The superior and inferior edge of the cup may be outlined by the circumlinear artery coursing round the rim.

The cup must be judged relative to the size of the disc. A modest amount of cupping may already herald loss of tissue in a small disc while a large amount of cupping may be physiologically normal in a large optic disc. The size of the disc leads to the greatest difficulties for observers judging the difference between physiological and pathological cupping. A large disc with a large cup will lead

many observers into a pathological call while a small disc with a modest but pathological cup may be overlooked as normal (Fig. 9.4).

An increase in the size of the cup may occur in two major ways: it may enlarge in a concentric fashion or in focal areas (Figs 9.5 and 9.6). The increase in the size of the cup is reflected in a uniform decrease in the neural rim around the cup.[5] There may be a generalised flattening of the usually convex structure of the disc particularly in small crowded discs, typically seen in hypermetropic eyes. This may be combined with a posterior bowing of the lamina cribrosa. There may be loss of tissue in any local area of the rim enlarging the cup only in that direction. If this is very focal and appears as if a bite has been taken from the inside of the rim it is termed a notch. If the tissue loss is more diffuse over a local area of the rim it would be termed an erosion of the rim. Both notching and erosions of the rim would be most commonly sited at the inferior and superior areas. These will both lead to an increase in the vertical cup/disc ratio and represent loss of axons from the arcuate areas of the retina which enter the poles of the optic disc. Optic disc defects such as this would be expected to produce a nasal step or an arcuate scotoma in the visual fields.

A notch or erosion of the rim may enlarge and ultimately is limited by the edge of the scleral canal marking the stage when virtually all neural tissue from that site has been lost.[5] A disc with a

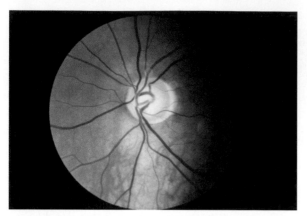

Fig. 9.5 Concentric pathological cupping of an optic disc. The C/D ratio is 0.7.

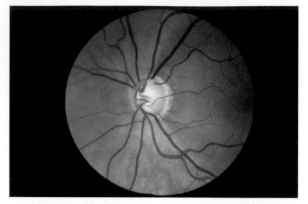

Fig. 9.6 Concentric enlargement of the cup but combined with pronounced focal erosion of the neural rim at the 12 o'clock position. There is a clearly visible retinal nerve fibre layer defect in the retina adjacent to the position of this notch.

concentric enlargement of the cup may continue to enlarge in this manner leading to an increasing cup-to-disc ratio in both vertical and horizontal directions. A disc with focal cupping is most likely to produce focal visual field defects whereas a cup with moderate concentric cupping is more likely to produce a visual field with a mixed picture of focal and diffuse loss. The focal notch is more common in normal tension glaucoma and may indicate a particular area of the disc in which the circulation has been compromised.

The most difficult morphological change in the disc structure to evaluate is a gentle concavity extending over most of the disc diameter. The edges of the cup are indiscernible as the slope is so gradual. The effect is like a saucer, hence the descriptive term saucerisation. This disc is also associated with glaucoma where the intraocular pressure may not seem unduly elevated but the patient is often elderly with systemic evidence of cardiovascular disease. Saucerisation of the disc is often overlooked using monocular disc examination and is more properly identified and evaluated by binocular examination.

An alteration in the configuration of the cup may be of pathological significance. The normal cup is a horizontal ovoid. The vertical cup-to-disc ratio would not normally be greater than the horizontal. If it is and the optic disc itself does not have an increased vertical diameter then this may signal pathological loss of neural rim. As already stated the rim is generally thickest in the inferior region followed by the superior, nasal and temporal rims

in order. If the inferior rim appears thin in comparison to the other rims, this may indicate early pathological change.

In evaluating the extent of the cup it is often useful to make a careful study of the rim at various sites and to estimate its thickness as a ratio relative to the disc diameter. The cup-to-disc ratio is inversely related to the 'rim-to-disc ratio'. Therefore assessment of the rim should lead to the cup-to-disc ratio by subtraction and will lead the observer to concentrate on a qualitative assessment of the neural tissue.

Both eyes tend to show symmetry of their disc size and degree of cupping unless there is a significant degree of anisometropia. Assuming an equal refractive status it would be unusual for there to be an asymmetry of 0.2 or greater in the cup-to-disc ratio between the two eyes. This is a particularly important sign in the earlier stages of glaucoma at which time it may be difficult to identify pathological signs in an individual disc with moderate cupping. In a patient with ocular hypertension and normal or equivocal visual field results this observation would imply an early glaucomatous process.

9.4.2 PALLOR

The base of the cup often appears pale in relation to the richer colour of the healthy neural rim. The lamina cribrosa is a tissue high in fibrous or glial content and is less vascular and more reflective, giving an appearance of pallor. The neural rim with a dense capillary network has a richer orange tinge to it. Pallor can be used as an illuminating sign showing the extent of the base of the cup but it is important to note that the region of pallor may not fully equate with the cup and may be a false localising sign. The contour of the rim should be used to evaluate the degree of cupping. However as the cup enlarges and there is a baring of the lamina cribrosa, there will be an apparent increase in pallor. Combined with this increase in pallor is an increased visibility of the pores through the lamina cribrosa. While increased numbers and size of these pores have been reported as signs of glaucoma, it is a poor and unreliable marker.

Pallor of the rim is a more subtle sign to detect and is of much greater pathological significance. The pallor will not be more prominent than that present in the base of the cup but it may be significantly paler than other areas of the neural rim. The pallor may also be more prominent if compared to the optic disc of the other eye. It may be combined with some degree of erosion of the rim. This combination of pallor and erosion makes identification of the rim contour and cup evaluation extremely difficult. A stereoscopic examination is most helpful in enabling an examiner to detect this. Pallor of the rim indicates focal damage to this region and will most probably be echoed by a visual field defect in the corresponding area.

Although pallor has been studied in both the rim and cup locations it is a very difficult finding to quantify. For the examiner it is an important qualitative sign to detect and it adds pathological significance to the cup configuration already quantified.[5]

9.5 VASCULAR SIGNS

9.5.1 OPTIC DISC HAEMORRHAGE

A haemorrhage on or around the optic disc is a common and important clinical sign (Fig. 9.7). The haemorrhage is most commonly seen as a small flame-shaped blotch on the neural rim extending over the disc margin onto the retina of

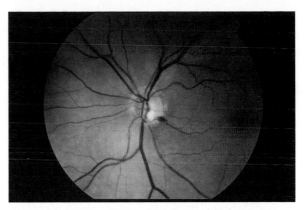

Fig. 9.7 This small optic disc illustrates several features. The disc seems small relative to the vessels entering it giving an impression of 'crowding'. There is a nerve fibre layer haemorrhage on the inferotemporal rim of the disc. The disc has a prominent notch of the neural rim inferiorly and the inferotemporal artery shows a focal narrowing just as it crosses the disc–retina junction.

the peripapillary region. It lies at the level of the retinal nerve fibre layer appearing superficial to the disc. This dictates its shape as it lies in and around bundles of nerve fibres streaming towards the scleral canal. The haemorrhage may also appear as a more rounded blot on the neural rim and this signifies its deeper position in the neural tissue. This would not generally cross the peripapillary border. It is unusual to find a haemorrhage within the cup itself as they are more common on the neural rim or peripapillary retina.

The haemorrhage may be most easily seen with a direct ophthalmoscope as this produces a higher magnification than most other techniques. The haemorrhage is particularly visible in red-free light, showing as a dark area. They can usually be identified by their ragged and feathered shape but a small haemorrhage may be difficult to distinguish from a small arteriole emerging from deeper tissues. The differentiation may only be apparent when the patient is examined at subsequent visits to see if a potential haemorrhage has disappeared or not.

Haemorrhages most commonly occur around the superior or inferior temporal poles of the optic disc, the areas most prone to glaucomatous excavation of the disc, however they can occur at any site. A haemorrhage takes between 6 weeks and 9 months to clear and if haemorrhage is repeatedly noted at a particular site it may be more likely to be a repeated event rather than slow resolution of the first. The site of the haemorrhage should be clearly documented; it may represent a marker for future pallor, notching, a retinal nerve fibre defect and subsequent visual field defects in a corresponding site. This may be up to several years after a haemorrhage has been noted.[6]

Although they are best known for their association with normal tension glaucoma haemorrhages may also occur in primary open angle glaucoma (with elevated intraocular pressure) and ocular hypertension. Their prevalence in these diseases can be compared as: normal tension glaucoma > primary open angle glaucoma > ocular hypertension > normal.[6] Optic disc haemorrhages may occur in patients with no identifiable pathology but this is uncommon.

The pathogenesis of the haemorrhage is unknown. It is probably a localised vascular crisis but whether this is initiated by a mechanical force related to intraocular pressure or if it is secondary to an ischaemic process such as reduced perfusion or local autoregulatory dysfunction is unknown. The presence of a haemorrhage certainly implies dysfunction at a microvascular level. As pathological damage may be detectable at the same site at a later date, the haemorrhage seems to be the earliest marker of potential microvascular decompensation at a particular site. Studies have also shown that there is a greater prevalence of disc haemorrhages in patients with progressive glaucoma. For this reason a patient with supposedly controlled intraocular pressure who is seen to have a further disc haemorrhage should be followed closely, as it may be a marker of progressive disease.

9.5.2 NASALISATION, BAYONETING AND BARING OF THE CIRCUMLINEAR VESSEL

The central retinal vessels emerge in the centre of the optic disc and initially lie opposed to the nasal wall of the cup. As cupping increases, the nasal rim is eroded and the nasal wall of the cup lies more distant from the centre of the disc. The vessels follow the erosion of the nasal wall and so appear to have been displaced nasally. This is termed nasal-

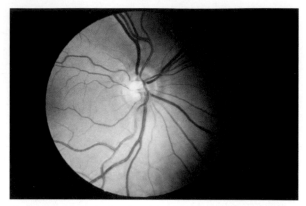

Fig. 9.8 There is focal erosion of the superior neural rim. This gives the impression that the rim has moved away from the circumlinear vessel. This is so-called 'baring of the circumlinear vessel'.

isation of the vessels. It is a non-specific and unquantifiable sign of glaucoma. It represents a moderate degree of tissue loss from an optic disc.

As the vessels ascend the sloping wall of the cup they pass over the rim of the cup to lie on the neural rim before passing onto the retina. In a healthy disc with a gently sloping cup this leads to a mild kink or change of direction in the vessel as it passes over the rim. If glaucomatous excavation of the disc is severe there may be an apparent loss of tissue extending underneath the neural rim. As a vessel 'disappears' into this recess and then suddenly reappears, it climbs over the rim at a point slightly lateral to its disappearance. This has the appearance of a bayonet with an apparent Z bend. This is termed bayoneting and is a sign of significant erosion of neural tissue and therefore quite advanced glaucoma. Both nasalisation and bayoneting are qualitative signs which would have been of more significance in the era where quantification of changes was not so paramount.

If there is localised erosion of the neuroretinal rim, the circumlinear vessel may be seen to have space between it and the rim against which it was assumed to previously lie. This effect is termed baring of the circumlinear vessel and may signify local erosion of the neural rim (Fig. 9.8).

9.5.3 LOCAL VASCULAR CHANGES

In advanced glaucoma there may be marked atrophy of the retinal nerve fibre layer and this is echoed by gross cupping of the optic disc. In this situation the retinal arterioles appear to be diffusely narrowed. The degree of narrowing is inversely related to the area of neural rim remaining. This change is probably an autoregulatory down grading of the circulation to the retinal circulation which subsequent to neural atrophy has a reduced metabolic need.

More localised narrowing of vessels may also be visible in the peripapillary region (see Fig. 9.7), especially with more advanced disease, and they correspond to areas of the disc that have increased cupping and peripapillary atrophy. They may again be as a result of reduced metabolic need in this focal area. Alternatively they may result from locally released vasoactive agents that cause an active local vasoconstriction. These vascular changes are further markers of pathological damage; they are uncommon in a normal situation.[7]

9.6 PERIPAPILLARY ATROPHY

The junctional zone between the retina, with underlying choroid and sclera, and the optic nerve is often poorly defined. A thin rim of sclera, Elschnig's ring, may surround the optic nerve and appears as a thin white rim to the pinker optic disc. Peripheral to this there may be areas usually concentric to the disc where the retina and choroid do not appear to extend directly to the disc edge but stop short. This may be a congenital finding or as part of a myopic fundus where the layers do not extend as far as the disc edge. This situation is often marked by a pigmented crescent. The pigment represents a folding of the retinal pigment epithelium and marks the area of misalignment of the layers in this region. With increased glaucomatous damage there is also an apparent increase in the prevalence of peripapillary atrophy and with more advanced damage there is an increase in the area of the peripapillary atrophy. The presence of the atrophy and its extent also relates to the presence and degree of cupping in the same area. Peripapillary atrophy is a further marker of damage in the peripapillary region.[8]

9.7 CLINICAL PERFORMANCE: A COMPLETE DISC EXAMINATION AND DOCUMENTATION

The disc should be evaluated with the direct or hand-held lens to an extent that the examiner feels confident in describing the contours and features apparent. This may require a combination of instruments and pupillary dilation. In a screening environment a decision must be taken in assessing whether any of the features present may indicate loss of neural tissue and therefore suspected glaucoma. This decision should be taken in an unbiased manner and not in relation to the level of intraocular pressure. If visual field examination has been carried out and suggests a defect then, if this is to be attributed to glaucoma as opposed to some other pathology such as retinal or neurological, changes will usually be apparent on the disc that correspond to the field defect. With the amount of redundancy in the visual system it appears that there is likely to be loss of tissue (cupping) before there is loss of function (fields). The early glaucoma patient is more likely to be detected by disc examination, as significant visual field defects are likely to represent a more moderate stage of the disease.

In a glaucoma management situation there may be a different approach to the examination. The disc features and size should have been previously documented. The task is then to assess whether there has been any change in the disc. At a basic level this would entail a judgement as to whether there has been a change in the cup-to-disc ratio. This can be easy to judge in a photographic series taken over many years but is difficult in shorter-term review when only basic information such as a cup/disc ratio is available. In a shared care environment the previous images must be studied and the disc examined to compare with the previous image and then any change documented. Most importantly specific features such as an optic disc haemorrhage or early notching should be examined for at each visit.

9.8 OPTIC NERVE IMAGING

As described, the optic disc and retinal nerve fibre layer are usually evaluated and documented by means of subjective techniques (drawings from ophthalmoscopy and monoscopic photographs). The ability to distinguish between normal and pathological is clearly based on the examiner's experience. A shared care scheme managing patients with ocular hypertension or the suspicion of glaucoma should have as a starting point an image of the optic disc.

In recent years advancing technologies have provided various imaging modalities to produce digital images of the optic nerve head (ONH) and the retinal nerve fibre layer (RNFL). They introduce quantitative and reproducible objective measurements of the optic disc and its surround that should improve the ability to discriminate normal from abnormal (glaucomatous) disease. Some of the devices measure a variety of optic disc parameters, whereas others are designed to measure only the thickness of the RNFL, or the whole retina. The information these methods provide is becoming an essential part of the management of patients with established glaucoma and also in that of patients who are glaucoma suspects and ocular hypertensives.

9.8.1 OPTIC NERVE HEAD STEREOSCOPIC COLOUR PHOTOGRAPHS

An optic nerve head stereoscopic colour photograph provides a high-resolution image of the optic disc and peripapillary retina. It creates a permanent record for close evaluation and future comparisons to detect optic disc glaucomatous progression. Provided that the stereo image base separation remains the same at each follow-up examination, changes in deepening and excavation of the cup can be observed over time. A dilated pupil and clear media are also required to give consistency in photograph quality.

The Discam (Marcher Enterprises Ltd, Hereford, England) is a dedicated stereoscopic optic disc camera. The stereo images provide an excellent high magnification stable picture for evaluation. With new software available, magnification corrected measurements can now be made. Despite excellent images, evaluation of photographs is still subjective. Several studies show that there is interobserver and intraobserver variability

in ONH assessment for detecting change over time in glaucoma and ocular hypertension even in a setting of highly trained glaucoma experts.[9,10]

9.8.2 CONFOCAL SCANNING LASER OPHTHALMOSCOPY

Confocal scanning laser ophthalmoscopes allow real-time three-dimensional topographic analysis of the optic disc and retina. The use of confocal optics, with minimum depth of focus, provides the ability to obtain good quality monochromatic images and reduces the need for pupil dilation and clear media. It provides rapid and reproducible measurements of optic disc surface height map (topography) on a pixel-by-pixel basis, as well as a reproducible analysis of various optic disc parameters. These include cup area, cup shape, disc area, maximum cup depth, cup volume, cup-to-disc area ratio, neuroretinal rim volume and neuroretinal rim area. An observer outlines the margin of the optic disc and a reference plane is positioned parallel to the surface and set below the surface. Structures above the reference plane are denoted as neuroretinal rim and the space below is denoted as optic cup.

The Heidelberg Retina Tomograph (HRT) (Heidelberg Engineering GmbH) has been widely investigated to assess the reproducibility of topographic measures and their clinical validity in differentiating normal from glaucomatous optic discs.[11] It is a powerful optic disc imaging technique because it provides a three-dimensional reconstruction of the retinal surface and optic cup supported by quantitative measurements, thus improving the follow-up of patients over time. The last few years have seen attempts to increase its diagnostic precision and hence the evolution of the HRT II which includes software that allows statistical analysis to facilitate longitudinal study aimed at better discrimination between normal and abnormal optic discs.[12] The software analyses the disc by segments and compares it with a database of normal values. The comparison is based on disc size and a probability map is produced indicating whether the disc is normal (Fig. 9.9a) or abnormal (Fig. 9.9b).

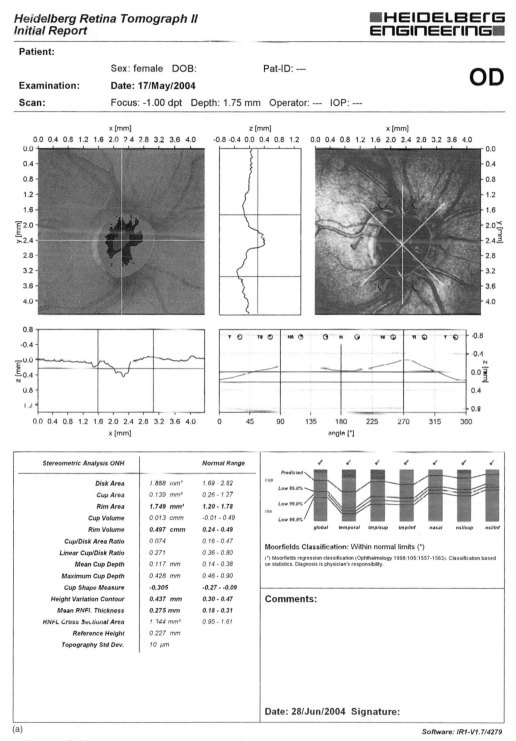

Fig. 9.9a The Moorfields Regression Analysis shows the ratio of the rim area compared to the disc area in six sectors and graphically presents the status of an individual optic nerve head in relation to normal eyes. Glaucomatous progression can also be quantified and displayed to show the trend over time. An example that falls within normal limits.

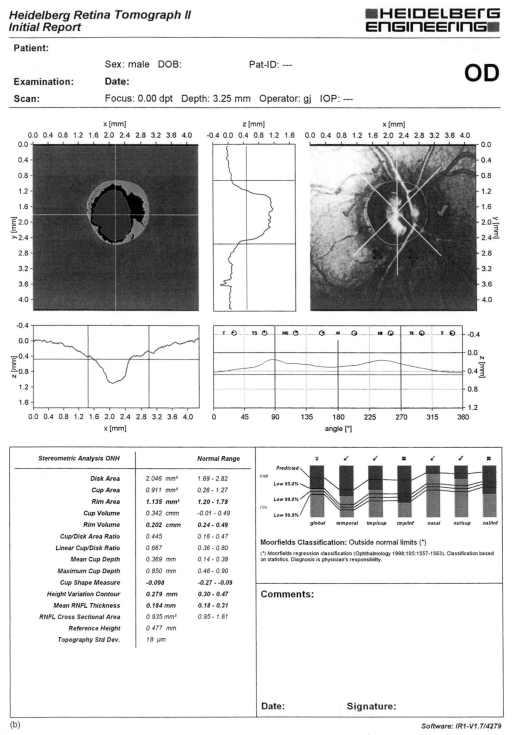

Fig. 9.9b The Moorfields Regression Analysis shows the ratio of the rim area compared to the disc area in six sectors and graphically presents the status of an individual optic nerve head in relation to normal eyes. Glaucomatous progression can also be quantified and displayed to show the trend over time. An example that falls outside normal limits.

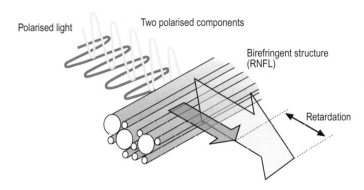

Fig. 9.10 Scanning laser polarimetry utilises polarised light to scan the back of the eye. The polarised light is made up of two orthogonal components. When these components pass through the retinal nerve fibre layer (RNFL; a birefringent medium), one component is changed. This change called retardation is then detected by an analyser. The amount of retardation from the RNFL is directly proportional to RNFL thickness.

9.8.3 SCANNING LASER POLARIMETRY

This technique performs polarised scans of the fundus building up a monochromatic image. This gives an assessment of the structure and thickness of the RNFL. Polarised light double passes through the RNFL and is split into two orthogonally polarised phase shifted components. (Fig. 9.10) Scanning laser polarimetry measures the phase shift (retardation) caused by the birefringent properties of the RNFL. Retardation has been shown to be linearly related to the thickness of the RNFL. The GDx VCC (Laser Diagnostic Technologies Inc.) is the most commercially up-to-date machine available and is marketed on the basis of a proprietary incorporated variable corneal compensator that eliminates corneal birefringence.[18] Scan acquisition time is 0.7 seconds.

The examination can be performed through an undilated pupil and does not require an entirely clear medium. A baseline image is automatically created from at least two scans. The optic disc margin is approximated on the image by a circle or ellipse that is placed by trained operators. The resultant printout displays the fundus image (a reflective image that is generated from the light reflected directly back), a RNFL thickness map (the map of retardation values), the TSNIT graph (the graph of RNFL thickness in the temporal, superior, nasal, inferior and temporal quadrants) which is characteristically a 'double hump' in normal cases. The software automatically calculates several RNFL parameters and displays them in a colour-coded table based on the probability of abnormality and classifies the RNFL thickness as 'within normal limits', 'borderline' or 'outside normal limits' (Figs 9.11 and 9.12). Globally and by quadrant these RNFL measures can be interpreted in one examination and compared over time.

9.8.4 OPTICAL COHERENCE TOMOGRAPHY

An optical coherence tomographer is a diagnostic precision imaging device providing scans that give cross-sectional images of the microstructure in ocular tissues, for a variety of posterior segment pathologies, to evaluate the layers within the retina. It uses an optical measurement known as low-coherence interferometry. The principle is similar to ultrasound, except light rather than sound is used.

The OCT 3 (Zeiss Humphrey Systems) performs a linear scan on the retina with a near infrared (low coherence) light beam with a depth resolution of <10 μm. The scan is acquired in approximately 1 second through a dilated pupil. A 4 mm radial line scan gives volumetric analysis of the optic nerve head and objectively finds the margin of the disc and volume of the cup. A circular scan centred on the optic disc in the peripapillary retina can be selected for RNFL measurements. RNFL thickness measurements are automatically displayed as two maps of retinal nerve fibre thickness around the optic disc. One map shows average RNFL thickness in micrometres, and the other shows RNFL thickness using a colour code that can be used for comparisons at follow-up examinations (Figs 9.13 and 9.14).

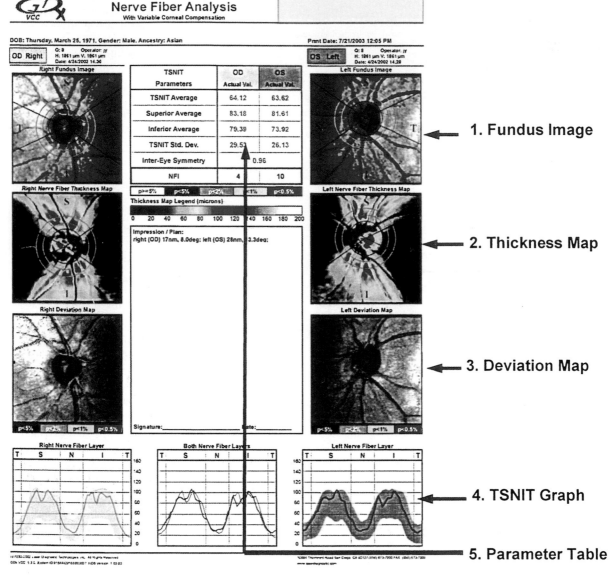

Fig. 9.11 Scanning laser polarimetry printout of a normal example.

Moderate Glaucoma Example

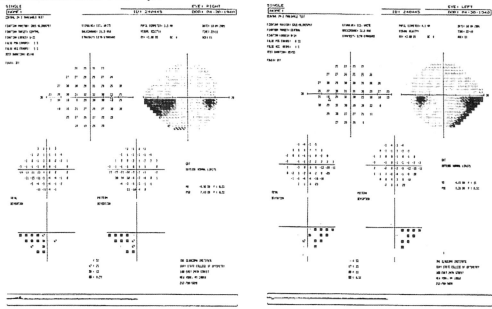

The Visual Fields for this patient show a clear nasal step inferiorly for both eyes.

1. Fundus Image
- Well focused
- Evenly illuminated
- Well centered

2. Thickness Map
- RNFL thinning Superior OU

3. Deviation Map
- Extensive RNFL loss in Superior OU

4. TSNIT Graph
- Falls outside shaded area (abnormal) in Superior region OU

5. Parameter Table
- Abnormal TSNIT Average OU
- Abnormal Superior Average OU
- NFI abnormal OU

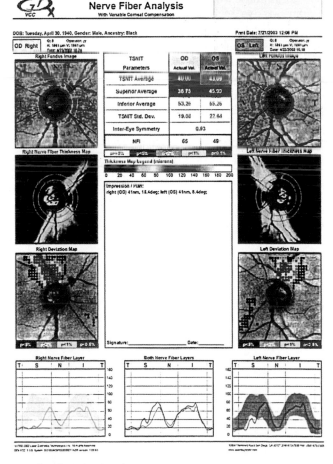

Fig. 9.12 Scanning laser polarimetry printout of an example of moderate glaucoma.

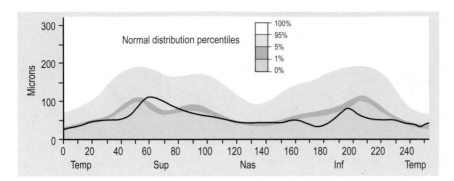

Fig. 9.13 Optical coherence tomography obtains measurements of retinal nerve fibre layer thickness along circular scans performed around the optic disc.

9.9 SUMMARY

The optic disc and the RNFL are the principal sites of apparent glaucomatous damage which may precede glaucomatous visual field alterations. It therefore seems appropriate to study these areas by means of clinical observation and the use of instrumentation capable of detecting early and late glaucomatous change. Thorough and expert examination of the disc and RNFL must form the central part of an assessment for glaucoma. The normal anatomy of the disc and its variations, in addition to optic disc size and its relationship to cupping, must be well understood so as to correctly identify glaucomatous change and not lead a patient into unnecessary anxiety and long-term investigation for a condition that they may not have. The utility of the described imaging techniques in isolation and in combination for the detection of early to moderate glaucomatous optic neuropathy requires further study.

Future work will determine an optimal testing strategy that is clinically practical. At this time none of these instruments alone is sufficient for the diagnosis and management of glaucoma.[14] The data they provide should be used only to complement the clinical picture available for the individual patient. It is also crucial to understand the relationship between the optic disc and visual field defects so that when field changes are identified they can be appropriately attributed to known patterns of glaucomatous damage at the optic disc or to retinal or neurological pathology elsewhere. To achieve a high sensitivity and specificity in the diagnosis, a practitioner should consider the disc on its own and then in relation to the visual field findings and vice versa. The intraocular pressure only then becomes relevant as a potential risk factor. As with so many art forms the more an optic disc is studied the more information will be obtained and the more confidence will be built around this central pivot for a diagnosis of glaucoma.

Scan Type:	Fast Optic Disc OD
Scan Date:	/2005
Scan Length:	4.0 mm

DOB: , ID:

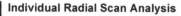

Individual Radial Scan Analysis

Rim Area (Vert.Cross Section):	0.042 mm²
Avg Nerve Width @ Disk	0.25 mm
Disk Diameter:	1.75 mm
Cup Diameter:	1.25 mm
Rim Length (Horiz.):	0.5 mm

Cup Offset (microns):

150

Signal Strength (Max 10)	7

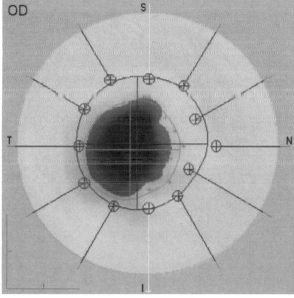

Optic Nerve Head Analysis Results

Vert. Integrated Rim Area (Vol.)	0.133 mm³
Horiz. Integrated Rim Width (Area)	1.394 mm²
Disk Area	2.517 mm²
Cup Area	1.353 mm²
Rim Area	1.164 mm²
Cup/Disk Area Ratio	0.538
Cup/Disk Horiz. Ratio	0.73
Cup/Disk Vert. Ratio	0.743

Plot Background:

☐ None   ☐ Absolute   ☑ Aligned and Shaded

Cup Offset for Topo (microns):	150
Cup Area (Topo):	1.132 mm²
Cup Volume (Topo):	0.271 mm³

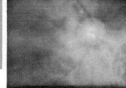

SCAN 1 : Results not Saved.
SCAN 2 : Results not Modified.
SCAN 3 : Results not Modified.
SCAN 4 : Results not Modified.
SCAN 5 : Results not Modified.
SCAN 6 : Results not Modified.

Signature:

Physician:

Fig. 9.14   Optical coherence tomography images of the optic nerve head in a glaucomatous eye.

References

1. Varma R, Tielsch JM, Quigley HA, et al. Race-, age-, gender-, and refractive error-related differences in the normal optic disc. Arch Ophthalmol 1994; 112:1068–1076.

2. Minckler DS. The organization of nerve fibre bundles in the primate optic nerve head. Arch Ophthalmol 1980; 98:1630.

3. Armaly MF. The optic cup in the normal eye. I. Cup width, depth, vessel displacement, ocular tension and outflow facility. Am J Ophthalmol 1969; 68:401.

4. Lim CS, O'Brien C, Bolton NM. A simple method to measure the optic disc size in glaucoma. J Glaucoma 1996; 5:4241–4245.

5. Jonas JB, Wido MB, Panda-Jonas S. Ophthalmoscopic evaluation of the optic nerve head. Surv Ophthalmol 1999; 43:293–320.

6. Airakinen J, Mustonen E, Alanko HI. Optic disc haemorrhages. Arch Ophthalmol 1981; 99:1795–1801.

7. Rankin SJA, Drance SM. Peripapillary focal retinal arteriolar narrowing in open angle glaucoma. J Glaucoma 1996; 5:22–28.

8. Primrose J. Early signs of the glaucomatous disc. Br J Ophthalmol 1971; 55:820–825.

9. Varma R, Steinmann WC, Scott IU. Expert agreement in evaluating the optic disc for glaucoma. Ophthalmology 1992; 99:215–221.

10. Tielsh JM, Katz J, Quigley HA, et al. Interobserver and intraobserver agreement in measurement of optic disc characteristics. Ophthalmology 1988; 95:350–356.

11. Kruse FE, Burk RO, Volck HE, et al. Reproducibility of topographic measurements of the optic nerve head with laser tomographic scanning. Ophthalmology 1989; 96:1320–1324.

12. Miglior S, Guareschi M, Vavassori M, et al. Detection of glaucomatous visual field changes using the Moorfields regression analysis of the Heidelberg retina tomograph. Am J Ophthalmol 2003; 136:26–33.

13. Weinreb R, Bowd C, Zangwill LM. Glaucoma detection using scanning laser polarimetry with variable corneal polarization compensation. Arch Ophthalmol 2002; 120:218–224.

14. Greaney M, Hoffman DC, Garway Heath DF, et al. Comparison of optic nerve imaging methods to distinguish normal eyes from those with glaucoma. Invest Ophthalmol Vis Sci 2002; 43:140–145.

Chapter 10

Medical management of the glaucomas 1: pharmacological principles

Jill Bloom

CHAPTER CONTENTS

10.1 THE HUMAN NERVOUS SYSTEM

The human nervous system comprises the central nervous system (CNS) and the peripheral nervous system (Fig. 10.1). The CNS consists of the brain and spinal cord. The peripheral nervous system is made up of afferent (sensory) nerve fibres which transmit impulses towards the CNS, and efferent (motor) nerve fibres which transmit impulses away from the CNS.

The efferent fibres can be further divided into somatic and autonomic nerve fibres (Fig. 10.2). Somatic nerve fibres are under voluntary control and send impulses from the CNS to voluntary (striated) muscle. Autonomic nerve fibres send impulses to organs which are not under voluntary control. These include the heart, bronchioles, gut, blood vessels and the glands which produce sweat and digestive, nasal, bronchial and lacrimal secretions. The autonomic nervous system is divided into the sympathetic and parasympathetic nervous systems.

10.2 THE AUTONOMIC NERVOUS SYSTEM

Many of the compounds used in the medical management of glaucoma exert their actions by modulating the activity of the autonomic nervous system. Therefore it is important to understand the basic principles underlying this system (Fig. 10.3).

10.2.1 NEUROTRANSMISSION

An impulse travels along the pre-ganglionic neurone, causing the release of a specific transmitter substance (also known as a neurohumoral transmitter) from vesicles at the end of the pre-ganglionic neurone into the synapse. The transmitter then combines with receptor sites on the cell body of the post-ganglionic neurone. This leads to a chain of events which results in an impulse being conducted along the post-ganglionic neurone. A specific transmitter is released from the vesicles at the end of this neurone into the neuro-effector synapse. The transmitter diffuses across this synapse and combines with receptor sites on the effector cell to bring about a change, i.e. contraction, relaxation or secretion.

10.2.2 NEUROHUMORAL TRANSMITTERS

■ Acetylcholine is the transmitter which is released from the **pre-ganglionic** neurones in both the sympathetic and the parasympathetic nervous systems.
■ Noradrenaline is the transmitter which is released from the **post-ganglionic** neurone in the sympathetic system (although there are some exceptions, i.e. transmission to the sweat glands).

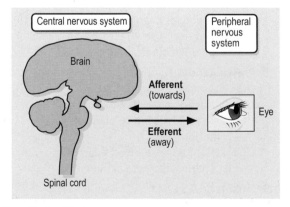

Fig. 10.1   The human nervous system.

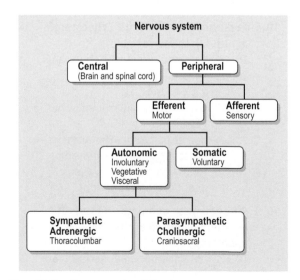

Fig. 10.2   Components of the human nervous system.

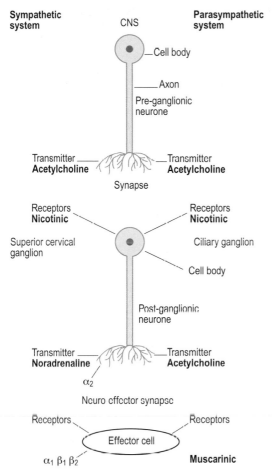

Fig. 10.3 Schematic representation of autonomic neurotransmission in the central nervous system (CNS).

■ Acetylcholine is the transmitter which is released from the **post-ganglionic** neurone in the parasympathetic system.

10.2.3 RECEPTORS

A variety of receptors is found in the autonomic nervous system. The main classes are: nicotinic, muscarinic, α_1, α_2, β_1 and β_2 receptors (Table 10.1). These receptors may be distinguished by their location within the autonomic nervous system and their ability to interact with either noradrenaline or acetylcholine. There are receptors which fit the shape of the acetylcholine molecule and receptors which fit the shape of the noradrenaline molecule (similar to a key fitting into a lock;

Fig. 10.4). Specific receptors, locations, and actions need to be acknowledged to explain some of the pharmacological effects of medications used in the management of glaucoma.

- α_1, α_2, β_1 and β_2 are found within the sympathetic system and interact with noradrenaline (although noradrenaline has a low affinity for β_2 receptors).
- α_1 receptors are mainly located on smooth muscle in the vasculature, and stimulation tends to cause smooth muscle contraction.
- α_2 receptors are mainly pre-synaptic receptors, and stimulation inhibits further release of noradrenaline.
- β_1 receptors are predominantly found in the heart and stimulation increases heart rate.
- β_2 receptors are mainly located on smooth muscle in the lung and vasculature, and stimulation tends to cause smooth muscle relaxation.
- Muscarinic receptors are located on the effector cells in the parasympathetic system and interact with acetylcholine which is released from the post-ganglionic neurones. Five subtypes of muscarinic receptor have been identified and these are known as M_1 to M_5. M_3 receptors are the subtypes most likely to be found in the eye, but for the purposes of this chapter the subtypes will not be distinguished.
- Nicotinic receptors interact with acetylcholine and are found on the cell bodies within the autonomic ganglia in both the sympathetic and the parasympathetic system. They are also found on skeletal (voluntary) muscle.

As a generalisation, stimulation of the sympathetic nervous system prepares the body for fear, fight or flight. The parasympathetic system is mainly concerned with digestion, secretion and the conservation of energy.

A number of the drugs used in the management of glaucoma target α, β or muscarinic receptor sites by competing with the transmitter, or affecting the concentration of transmitter in the neuro-effector

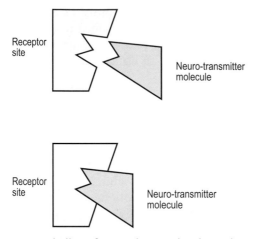

Fig. 10.4 Binding of transmitter molecule at the receptor site. The transmitter molecule must be shaped so that it can fit into the receptor site. Top, transmitter molecule approaches receptor site; bottom, transmitter molecule binds with receptor.

synapse. One of the primary aims in glaucoma management is to lower the intraocular pressure (IOP) in patients with raised pressures, to a level which prevents further visual damage. IOP is controlled by the rate of aqueous humour formation in the ciliary processes and the rate of outflow from the eye. Outflow may be conventional, via the anterior chamber, trabecular meshwork, canal of Schlemm and into the general venous circulation, or non-conventional (uveoscleral) through the ciliary muscle, into the suprachoroidal space, sclera and orbit. Drug therapy tends to focus on lowering raised IOP, therefore it is necessary to know the location and action of the ocular autonomic receptors (Table 10.2).

The European Glaucoma Society 'Terminology and Guidelines for Glaucoma 2003' advocates the use of target pressures (see Chapter 11).[1] These target pressures will vary between individuals depending upon risk factors. They are in the order of a 20–40% reduction of the initial IOP at which damage occurred.

Table 10.1 Location of and actions associated with sympathetic and parasympathetic receptors in the autonomic nervous system

	Receptors	Main location	Action due to stimulation (some examples)
Sympathetic/adrenergic	Nicotinic	Cell bodies within autonomic ganglia	Depolarisation of post-ganglionic neurone
	α_1	Effector cell	Arterioles: constrict; blood pressure increases; skin goes paler due to vasoconstriction Bladder sphincter: constricts Blood glucose: increases
	α_2	Presynaptic	Inhibits noradrenaline release from pre-synaptic vesicles
	β_1	Effector cell	Heart: rate increases
	β_2	Effector cell	Bronchial muscle: relaxes and dilates bronchioles Blood glucose: increases
Parasympathetic/cholinergic	Nicotinic	Cell bodies within autonomic ganglia	Depolarisation of post-ganglionic neurone
	Muscarinic	Effector cell	Glands secrete: salivary secretion; bronchial secretion; nasal secretion Heart: rate decreases Bladder: detrusor contracts (bladder empties) Digestive system: increases motility and tone; sphincters relax; secretion increases

Table 10.2   Ocular autonomic receptors

Eye effector cell	Sympathetic/adrenergic receptors (stimulation)	Parasympathetic/cholinergic receptors (stimulation)
Iris dilator	$\alpha_1 \rightarrow$ Mydriasis	
Iris sphincter		Muscarinic $\rightarrow$ Miosis
Ciliary muscle		Muscarinic $\rightarrow$ Accommodation
Epithelium of the ciliary processes	$\beta_2 \rightarrow \uparrow$ and $\downarrow$ aqueous formation	
Outflow channels	$\beta_2 \rightarrow \uparrow$ Outflow	
Outflow channels	$\alpha_1 \rightarrow \uparrow$ Outflow	
Blood vessels	$\alpha_1 \rightarrow$ Vasoconstriction	Muscarinic $\rightarrow$ Vasodilatation
Blood vessels	$\beta_2 \rightarrow$ Vasodilatation	
Lacrimal gland		Muscarinic $\rightarrow$ Secretion
Müller's muscle	$\alpha_1 \rightarrow$ Constriction (lid retraction)	

Table 10.3   Pressure-lowering effects of drug classes

Drug class	Approximate intraocular pressure reduction (%)
Prostaglandin $F_{2\alpha}$ analogues	30–25
β-blockers (except betaxolol)	25–20
α_2-agonists	25–20
Parasympathomimetics (pilocarpine)	25–20
Carbonic anhydrase inhibitors (oral—acetazolamide)	25–20
β-blockers (betaxolol)	20–15
Carbonic anhydrase inhibitors (topical)	20–15
Adrenoceptor agonists (dipivefrine)	20–15

Monotherapy is recommended but in practice most patients will eventually require several different types of glaucoma medication. Presently, the majority of ophthalmologists in the UK use either β-blockers and/or prostaglandin $F_{2\alpha}$ analogues as first-line therapy. Table 10.3 gives approximate pressure-lowering effects of the various drug classes.

10.3 β-ADRENOCEPTOR ANTAGONISTS (β-BLOCKERS)

10.3.1 ASSUMED PRINCIPAL ACTION

They lower IOP by blocking β-receptors located on the human ciliary epithelium of the ciliary processes, thereby reducing aqueous humour formation. Many β-blocking drugs are available, but only a few are used in ophthalmology (Table 10.4). The differences between the various β-blockers are due to:

■ Their intrinsic sympathomimetic activity (ISA) or partial agonist activity. Carteolol is the only topical β-blocker which possesses ISA (Table 10.5). When one considers a scale, where one end of the scale represents a drug with 100% receptor blocking activity (antagonist) and the other end represents 100% receptor stimulating activity (agonist), there will be points along the scale near the antagonist end where the drug may be considered to have mainly antagonist activity but also possess a small amount of agonist activity (ISA). This may be important when considering the adverse effect of β-blocker eye drops in relation to the slowing of the heart (bradycardia). If a patient with a normal heart rate is started on a β-blocker without ISA and subsequently develops bradycardia, theoretically carteolol may be the β-blocker of choice, assuming that the heart rate does not fall significantly, in which case the drug should be stopped and an alternative non-β-blocking drug found.

■ Their selectivity: (i) ability to block predominantly β_1 receptors (cardioselective) and (ii) ability to block both β_1 and β_2 receptors (non-selective). Timolol, carteolol, levobunolol, and metipranolol block both β_1 and β_2 receptors and are referred to as non-selective, whereas betaxolol blocks predominantly β_1 receptors and is referred to as cardioselective. The β_1 selectivity of betaxolol does not explain why it should lower IOP although several explanations have been put forward. One theory suggests that at high concentrations, these drugs lose their selectivity and block both β_1 and β_2 receptors.[2]

■ Ability to block α receptors. It is generally accepted that the ophthalmic β-blockers do not have any significant α blocking activity.

■ Membrane stabilising activity (resulting in corneal anaesthesia). It is generally accepted that the ophthalmic β-blockers have very little membrane-stabilising activity.

Table 10.4 β-blocking drugs used in ophthalmology

Drug	Commercial product
Timolol	Timoptol® 0.25% and 0.5% (preserved and unpreserved) Timoptol® LA 0.25% and 0.5% (gel-forming solution) (preserved) Generic 0.25% and 0.5% (preserved) Combigan® (timolol 0.5% with brimonidine 0.2%) (preserved) Cosopt® (timolol 0.5% with dorzolamide 2%) (preserved) Xalacom® (timolol 0.5% with latanoprost 0.005%) (preserved) Timolol 0.1% (gel) Nyogel® (preserved)
Betaxolol	Betoptic® suspension 0.25% (preserved and unpreserved) Betoptic® 0.5% (preserved)
Carteolol	Teoptic® 1% and 2% (preserved)
Levobunolol	Betagan® 0.5% (preserved and unpreserved)
Metipranolol	Metipranolol Minims® 0.1% and 0.3% (unpreserved)

Table 10.5 Differences in receptor activity and intrinsic sympathomimetic activity of β-blockers

Drug	Receptor blocked	Intrinsic sympathomimetic activity
Timolol	β_1 and β_2	No
Betaxolol	β_1	No
Carteolol	β_1 and β_2	Yes
Levobunolol	β_1 and β_2	No
Metipranolol	β_1 and β_2	No

- Lipophilicity (lipid solubility). Lipophilicity is important when considering penetration across the cornea. Theoretically, increased lipid solubility may also be responsible for CNS effects such as depression.

10.3.2 MANAGEMENT OF GLAUCOMA

β-blockers block the β_2 receptors on the epithelium of the ciliary processes and aqueous outflow channels, and are used in the management of primary open angle glaucoma, ocular hypertension and some secondary glaucomas. Dosages used are shown in Table 10.6 and the time of action in Table 10.7.

10.3.3 THEORY OF PHARMACOLOGICAL ACTION

Human ciliary processes contain predominantly β_2-adrenergic receptors.[3] It is debatable as to whether stimulation of β_2 receptors in the human ciliary epithelium causes increased or decreased aqueous formation. Research studies where the same β-agonist has been used have come to different conclusions.[4,5] However, it is accepted that blocking β_2 receptors results in decreased aqueous formation.[6]

It is possible that there are some β_2 receptors in the outflow channels, although conclusive evidence to demonstrate their existence in humans is lacking. It was deduced that these β_2 receptors exist, since the effect of increasing aqueous outflow produced by adrenaline (α_1-, α_2-, β_1- and β_2-agonist) was blocked by timolol (β_1- and β_2-blocker). One can therefore conclude that either β_1 or β_2 receptors are present in the outflow channels. Betaxolol (β_1-blocker), did not block this effect, further suggesting that it was the β_2 receptors which were present in the outflow channels.[7] These β_2 receptors do not have inherent activity as β-blocking drugs used alone have little or no effect on outflow facility.[8] The main effect of the β-blocking drugs is to reduce aqueous humour formation thereby lowering IOP.

All the drugs, with the exception of betaxolol, lower IOP by a similar amount. Betaxolol does not offer as great a lowering of IOP, but it is still a significant lowering.

Table 10.6 Dosage of β-blockers	
Drug	Dose
Timolol	One drop twice a day
Long-acting preparation	One drop once a day
Combigan®	One drop twice a day
Cosopt®	One drop twice a day
Xalacom®	One drop in the morning
Nyogel®	One drop once a day
Betaxolol	One drop twice a day
Carteolol	One drop twice a day
Levobunolol	One drop once or twice a day
Metipranolol	One drop twice a day

Table 10.7 Time of action of β-blockers			
Drug	Onset of lowering of IOP	Time to maximum lowering of IOP	Duration of IOP lowering effect
Timolol	Within 30 minutes	≈2 hours	≈24 hours
Betaxolol	Within 30 minutes	≈2 hours	≈12 hours
Carteolol	Within 1 hour	≈4 hours	12–24 hours
Levobunolol	Within 1 hour	2–6 hours	12–24 hours
Metipranolol	Within 30 minutes	≈2 hours	≈24 hours

Table 10.8 Parasympathomimetic drugs used in ophthalmology		
Drug	**Commercial product**	**Action**
Pilocarpine	Generic 0.5%, 1%, 2%, 3%, 4% (preserved) Minims® 2%, 4% (unpreserved) Pilogel® 4% (gel) (preserved)	Directly acting muscarinic agonist (Has actions similar to acetylcholine)
Carbachol	No longer available	Directly acting muscarinic agonist
Eserine/ physostigmine	No longer available	Indirectly acting agonist Reversibly blocks enzyme (acetylcholinesterase) which is responsible for acetylcholine breakdown
Echothiophate /phospholine iodide	Named patient only 0.125% (preserved)	Indirectly acting agonist Irreversibly blocks enzyme (acetylcholinesterase)

10.3.4 MAIN ADVERSE EFFECTS DUE TO PHARMACOLOGICAL ACTIONS

Ocular adverse effects

The prevalence of ocular adverse effects to topical β-blockers is low. β-blockers do not affect pupil size or accommodation, although there have been a few reports of decreased corneal sensitivity.

Systemic adverse effects

Systemic adverse effects of β-blockers focus on the effects of blocking β_1 receptors in the heart or blocking β_2 receptors on the smooth bronchial muscle of the lung. Blocking β_1 receptors may cause a reduction in heart rate, reduction in heart contractility, cardiac failure, arrhythmias, syncope and hypotension. These drugs are contraindicated in patients with sinus bradycardia (slow heart), second or third degree atrioventricular block (heart block), cardiac failure or cardiogenic shock.

Blocking β_2 receptors may impair respiratory function by causing constriction of the bronchioles resulting in wheezing, dyspnoea or bronchospasm. Non-selective β-blockers are contraindicated in patients with asthma or chronic obstructive pulmonary disease. Betaxolol is cardioselective and has less effect on respiratory function than the non-selective drugs. However, betaxolol must still be used with caution when given to patients with obstructive pulmonary disease.

The ophthalmic β-blockers are highly lipophilic and may cross the blood–brain barrier into the CNS. This may give rise to depression, fatigue, confusion, lethargy and hallucinations. These effects are rare, but have been reported in some patients.

10.4 PARASYMPATHOMIMETICS (CHOLINERGIC AGONISTS) (MIOTICS)

Miotics, which include pilocarpine (Table 10.8), are long-established medications with a good safety record and significant IOP lowering effects. Pilocarpine has been used in ophthalmology for over 100 years and is used in the management of both open angle glaucoma and relieving acute attacks of angle closure glaucoma (Table 10.9).

10.4.1 ASSUMED PRINCIPAL ACTION

Lowering IOP by stimulating muscarinic receptors on the ciliary smooth muscle, and thus opening the trabecular meshwork to increase aqueous humour outflow. Miotics are used in the management of primary open angle glaucoma (POAG), ocular hypertension, some secondary glaucomas and relieving acute angle closure attacks.

10.4.2 THEORY OF PHARMACOLOGICAL ACTION

Parasympathetic stimulation of the muscarinic receptors located on the longitudinal muscle fibres

Table 10.9   Dosage and time of action of parasympathomimetics

Drug	Dose	Onset of lowering of IOP	Time to maximum lowering of IOP	Duration of IOP lowering effect
Pilocarpine	One drop is usually instilled four times a day, but dose varies according to severity of disease, resulting IOP, and tolerance of adverse effects. Concentrations of pilocarpine above 4% seem to be of little value except in highly pigmented patients who require higher concentrations. It is believed that pilocarpine binds to pigment The ophthalmic gel is applied once daily at bedtime	Minutes	2–3 hours	≈5 hours

of the ciliary muscle produces a pull on the scleral spur, posteriorly and internally, which opens up the trabecular meshwork and leads to an increase in aqueous outflow.[9]

10.4.3 USE OF PARASYMPATHOMIMETICS IN POAG

The iris is not directly attached to the scleral spur or trabecular meshwork and constriction of the pupil does not play a principal part in the reduction of IOP. Miosis can be thought of as an unwanted effect in this process. These drugs may also theoretically hinder or reduce drainage by the unconventional (uveoscleral) outflow pathway, by contraction of the ciliary muscle, and obliterating the spaces between the muscle bundles.

10.4.4 USE OF PARASYMPATHOMIMETICS IN ACUTE ANGLE CLOSURE GLAUCOMA

In an acute angle closure attack, miotics do not have pressure lowering effects at very high IOPs, as the iris may become ischaemic and unresponsive. IOP should be brought down to about 30 mmHg by other drugs, such as intravenous acetazolamide, intravenous mannitol or oral glycerol, before the miotic drugs can exert their effect. The duration of lowering of IOP varies with the individual and the severity of the disease.

10.4.5 MAIN ADVERSE EFFECTS DUE TO PHARMACOLOGICAL ACTIONS

Pilocarpine has a good safety profile and does not produce serious adverse effects at normal doses. However, it does cause a number of annoying ocular effects. Many of these adverse effects are due to unwanted stimulation of muscarinic receptors at other sites, e.g. iris sphincter and blood vessels.

Ocular adverse effects

Ciliary spasm is one of the most troublesome effects of miotics. It is more pronounced in younger patients (under 50 years). Headaches and ciliary spasm tend to be more severe during the first two weeks of treatment. Vasodilatation of the conjunctival blood vessels occurs on instillation of miotic drugs resulting in hyperaemia, but this resolves after approximately 30 minutes. Miotics cause darkening or dimming of vision especially at night and patients may experience difficulty with night driving. If the patient has cataracts, the vision may be further impaired.

Soon after pilocarpine eye drops are instilled, the anterior chamber becomes shallower and the crystalline lens becomes axially thicker and moves forward. This is maximal at 45–60 minutes, then disappears after approximately 100 minutes.[10] On rare occasions, IOP may increase due to pupillary block. Sometimes the lens is so far forward that it touches the iris, and the pressure in the posterior chamber increases, pushing the iris forward at the periphery, causing blockage of the angle.[11]

Cholinergic miotics cause a breakdown in the blood–aqueous barrier and may allow entry of protein, cells or fibrin into the anterior chamber. Therefore cholinergic miotics should be avoided in patients with neovascular glaucoma, uveitic glaucoma or any condition where there is associated ocular inflammation. There is some circumstantial evidence that high myopes and patients with pre-existing peripheral retinal disease may be predisposed to retinal detachment. Some ophthalmologists believe that the cholinesterase enzyme inhibitors are more likely to be responsible for this than pilocarpine.

In patients with open angle glaucoma taking long-term miotic therapy, the eyes should be dilated once a year to prevent permanent miosis due to loss of tone in the iris dilator and fibrosis of the iris sphincter muscle.

Systemic adverse effects

Systemic toxicity from cholinergic miotics is rare at standard doses. On intensive use of pilocarpine eye drops in the management of angle closure attacks, systemic adverse effects such as sweating, salivation, nausea, vomiting, retching, tremor and hypotension have occurred.

10.5 ADRENOCEPTOR AGONISTS (ADRENERGIC AGONISTS: SYMPATHOMIMETIC AGONISTS)

10.5.1 ASSUMED PRINCIPAL ACTION

Lowering of IOP by increasing aqueous outflow facility.

Table 10.10 Adrenoceptor agonists and their receptor activity

Drug	Commercial product	Receptor stimulated
Adrenaline	No longer available	$\alpha_1, \alpha_2, \beta_1, \beta_2$
Dipivefrine	Propine® 0.1% (preserved)	$\alpha_1, \alpha_2, \beta_1, \beta_2$

10.5.2 MANAGEMENT OF GLAUCOMA

Adrenoceptor agonists are used in the management of primary open angle glaucoma and ocular hypertension.

10.5.3 THEORY OF PHARMACOLOGICAL ACTION

Adrenaline increases conventional aqueous humour outflow, uveoscleral outflow, and aqueous humour formation.[12,13] The mechanism of action of adrenaline is not understood. Adrenaline stimulates α_1, α_2, β_1, and β_2 receptors (Table 10.10). α_1 receptors are mainly post-synaptic and α_2 receptors are mainly pre-synaptic, but there are some post-synaptic α_2 receptors. Stimulation of α_2 receptors prevents further release of the transmitter noradrenaline from the nerve terminal (Fig. 10.5), and this can be thought of as a feedback mechanism. Most research papers examining the effects of adrenaline do not distinguish between the two types of α or β receptors.

Adrenaline has a variety of effects on aqueous humour dynamics, but at present it is believed that the most notable effects are those causing an increase in conventional aqueous humour outflow. This is believed to be mainly mediated by stimulation of β_2 receptors[4] and α receptors[12] in the outflow channels.

10.5.4 DIPIVEFRINE

Dipivefrine is a prodrug of adrenaline. Prodrugs are inactive compounds and need to be converted to active drug. Dipivefrine is lipophilic and therefore penetrates the cornea more effectively than adrenaline (Table 10.11). This means that a lower concentration can be used, which should

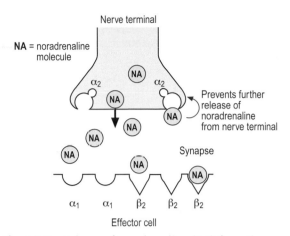

Fig. 10.5 Release of noradrenaline (NA) from the post-ganglionic neurone.

theoretically give rise to fewer adverse effects. Dipivefrine is converted to adrenaline by tissue enzymes in the eye.

10.5.5 MAIN ADVERSE EFFECTS DUE TO PHARMACOLOGICAL ACTIONS

Ocular adverse effects

Repeated vasoconstriction of the conjunctival blood vessels leads to a reactive hyperaemia which is a common side effect of these drugs. Unfortunately, after several years treatment, many patients experience allergic skin reactions and pigmentary deposits in the conjunctiva, cornea and eyelids. Soft contact lenses may also become discoloured.

Adrenaline or dipivefrine should not be used in aphakia as they give rise to macular oedema in this patient group. Many ophthalmologists believe that adrenaline and dipivefrine have an adverse effect on the conjunctiva and reduce the success rate of glaucoma surgery.

Systemic adverse effects

The most important adverse effects of the sympathomimetic drugs, adrenaline and dipivefrine, are those on the cardiovascular system. These include increased heart rate (tachycardia), palpitations and arrhythmias. Blood pressure may also increase due to the vasoconstrictive action of the adrenergic agonists. These drugs must be used with extreme caution in those patients with cardiovascular disease or hypertension.

Interactions

Systemic medications with sympathomimetic activity may potentiate these adverse effects, for example tricyclic antidepressants, such as amitriptyline or imipramine. Interaction with monoamine-oxidase inhibitors can cause a dangerous rise in blood pressure. Monoamine-oxidase inhibitors should be stopped for at least 2 or 3 weeks before the patient uses another drug with sympathomimetic action.

10.5.6 α$_2$-AGONISTS

Assumed principal action

Lowering of IOP by reducing aqueous humour formation.

Table 10.11	Dosage and time of action of adrenoceptor agonists			
Drug	Dose	Onset of lowering of IOP	Time to maximum lowering of IOP	Duration of IOP lowering effect
Adrenaline	One drop once or twice a day	Within 1 hour	≈4 hours	12–24 hours
Dipivefrine	One drop twice a day	≈30 minutes	≈1 hour	12–24 hours

Table 10.12 α₂ agonists and their receptor activity		
Drug	**Commercial product**	**Receptor stimulated**
Apraclonidine	Iopidine® 0.5% (preserved) Iopidine® 1% (unpreserved)	α_2
Brimonidine	Alphagan® 0.2% (preserved) Combigan® (timolol 0.5% with brimonidine 0.2%) (preserved)	α_2

Table 10.13 Dosage and time of action of α₂ agonists				
Drug	**Dose**	**Onset of lowering of IOP**	**Time to maximum lowering of IOP**	**Duration of IOP lowering effect**
Apraclonidine	One drop three times a day	1 hour	3–5 hours	12 hours
Brimonidine	One drop twice a day	Rapid	2 hours	12 hours

Management of glaucoma

Apraclonidine is indicated for short-term use in the management of chronic glaucoma in patients on maximum tolerated therapy who require additional IOP lowering to delay surgical or laser procedures. Brimonidine is indicated in the management of open angle glaucoma and ocular hypertension.

Theory of pharmacological action

Several theories exist as to how α_2-agonists exert their IOP lowering effects. These drugs also have slight activity on α_1 receptors, but brimonidine is far more selective for α_2 receptors than apraclonidine (Table 10.12). Stimulation of α_2 receptors prevents further release of the transmitter nora-drenaline into the synapse, and this in turn is thought to decrease aqueous humour formation. Brimonidine has also been shown to increase uveoscleral outflow,[14] whereas apraclonidine has not shown this effect. Apraclonidine is indicated for short-term use in the UK as the IOP-lowering effect usually diminishes over a period of approximately 4 weeks. However some patients may benefit for longer periods. Brimonidine, on the other hand, is licensed for long-term use and the IOP lowering is maintained in the majority of patients. This indicates that there must be other processes or receptors in existence which also regulate IOP. One theory which has been put forward is the existence of an imidazoline receptor[15] which may be involved in IOP regulation. Dosage and time of action are given in Table 10.13.

10.5.7 MAIN ADVERSE EFFECTS DUE TO PHARMACOLOGICAL ACTIONS

Ocular adverse effects

The most common effect seen with these drugs is conjunctival hyperaemia.

Systemic adverse effects

These drugs have minimal effects on the cardiovascular system, but caution must still be exercised when managing patients with cardiovascular disease.

Interactions

Interactions are the same as for those patients using either adrenaline or dipivefrine.

10.6 ADRENERGIC ANTAGONISTS (SYMPATHOLYTICS)

10.6.1 ASSUMED PRINCIPAL ACTION

Sympatholytics such as guanethidine cause depletion of stores of noradrenaline transmitter from vesicles inside the nerve terminal.

10.6.2 MANAGEMENT OF GLAUCOMA

Guanethidine has been used previously in the management of primary open angle glaucoma and secondary glaucoma (Table 10.14).

10.6.3 THEORY OF PHARMACOLOGICAL ACTION

Guanethidine initially displaces the transmitter noradrenaline from its storage vesicles inside the nerve terminal, giving rise to a transient increase in outflow facility and mydriasis. When the stores of noradrenaline are depleted, aqueous humour formation is reduced and the pupil becomes miosed.

10.6.4 MAIN ADVERSE EFFECTS DUE TO PHARMACOLOGICAL ACTIONS

The sympatholytic action of guanethidine causes depletion of noradrenaline transmitter, resulting in loss of stimulation to the iris dilator, which is no longer able to contract. The result is miosis. Maintenance of contraction of Müller's muscle is also lost and may result in lid ptosis. Concentrations greater than 5% are usually needed to cause lid ptosis.

10.7 CARBONIC ANHYDRASE INHIBITORS

10.7.1 ASSUMED PRINCIPAL ACTION

Lowering of IOP by blocking the enzyme carbonic anhydrase in the ciliary epithelial cells, thereby reducing aqueous humour formation.

10.7.2 MANAGEMENT OF GLAUCOMA

Carbonic anhydrase inhibitors (Table 10.15) are used in the management of primary open angle glaucoma and secondary glaucoma. Acetazolamide injection can be used in acute angle closure glaucoma. Brinzolamide can be used in ocular hypertension. Dorzolamide can also be used in ocular hypertension and pseudoexfoliative glaucoma.

10.7.3 THEORY OF PHARMACOLOGICAL ACTION

The mechanism by which carbonic anhydrase inhibitors reduce aqueous humour formation is not fully understood. Carbonic anhydrase is an enzyme found in the corneal endothelium, pigmented and non-pigmented ciliary epithelium, Müller's cells and retinal pigment epithelium. Blocking carbonic anhydrase in the ciliary

Table 10.14	Sympatholytics
Drug	**Commercial product**
Guanethidine	No longer available

Table 10.15	Carbonic anhydrase inhibitors and their dosages	
Drug	**Commercial product**	**Dose**
Acetazolamide	Diamox® 250 mg tablets Diamox® 250 mg slow release capsules Diamox® 500 mg injection	One tablet once to four times a day One capsule once or twice a day 250 mg to 1 g daily
Brinzolamide	Azopt® 1% eye drops (preserved)	One drop two or three times a day
Dorzolamide	Trusopt® 2% eye drops (preserved) Cosopt® (dorzolamide 2% with timolol 0.5%) (preserved)	Monotherapy: One drop three times a day With β-blocker: One drop twice a day

epithelium results in decreased aqueous formation. One theory which tries to explain this action is that within the cell a chemical reaction is taking place:

$$\text{Carbon dioxide + Water} \xrightleftharpoons[\text{anhydrase}]{\text{Carbonic}} \text{Carbonic acid} \Leftrightarrow \text{Bicarbonate ion + Hydrogen ion}$$

Bicarbonate ions are actively secreted from the ciliary epithelial cells into the posterior chamber, and sodium ions are also actively secreted with the bicarbonate. This causes an osmotic gradient which causes fluid to flow from the epithelial cells into the posterior chamber resulting in aqueous humour secretion. The enzyme carbonic anhydrase catalyses the reaction of the hydration of carbon dioxide to carbonic acid. Carbonic acid instantaneously dissociates into bicarbonate ions and hydrogen ions. Hydrogen ions produce an acidic environment. It can be seen from the reaction that if bicarbonate ions are lost from the cell, hydrogen ions remain, resulting in an acidic environment. To re-establish the equilibrium, carbonic anhydrase must catalyse the production of more carbonic acid and hence more bicarbonate. If this enzyme is blocked, the result is an acidic cell which can no longer secrete bicarbonate and aqueous production ceases.

There has been concern among some ophthalmologists regarding the long-term effects of potentially blocking the endothelial pump mechanism and thereby affecting corneal hydration. Hence these ophthalmologists do not use topical carbonic anhydrase inhibitors when the cornea is in a compromised state.

10.7.4 MAIN ADVERSE EFFECTS DUE TO PHARMACOLOGICAL ACTIONS

Acetazolamide acts as a diuretic during the first few weeks of treatment. This may cause polyuria (large volumes of urine) and potassium loss. These effects then gradually wear off. Patients complain of paraesthesia (tingling in the extremities, especially hands and feet), taste disturbance, headache and fatigue. Less common adverse effects are dizziness, tinnitus (buzzing or ringing in the ears), depression, gastrointestinal disturbances such as nausea and vomiting, blood dyscrasias, renal colic and calculi.

Since brinzolamide and dorzolamide are topical carbonic anhydrase inhibitors, less drug will be absorbed into the systemic circulation and therefore there is less chance of dose-related adverse effects. Some of these adverse effects are still seen in some patients. The commonest adverse effects with the topical carbonic anhydrase inhibitors are foreign body sensation, ocular hyperaemia and a bitter taste in the mouth.

Acetazolamide, brinzolamide and dorzolamide all have the chemical structure of a group of compounds known as sulphonamides and should not be used when the patient has a known sulphonamide allergy, as they may cause a rash and skin eruptions. Carbonic anhydrase inhibitors are contraindicated when sodium or potassium blood serum levels are depressed, especially in the case of kidney or liver failure.

10.8 PROSTAGLANDIN $F_{2\alpha}$ ANALOGUES

10.8.1 ASSUMED PRINCIPAL ACTION

Lowering IOP by increasing non-conventional (uveoscleral) outflow facility of aqueous humour.[16] It has been suggested that bimatoprost may also increase conventional trabecular outflow.

10.8.2 MANAGEMENT OF GLAUCOMA

Prostaglandin $F_{2\alpha}$ analogues (Table 10.16) are used in the management of open angle glaucoma and ocular hypertension.

10.8.3 THEORY OF PHARMACOLOGICAL ACTION

Prostaglandins are a group of compounds which occur naturally in the body and are synthesised following tissue injury. One of their main biological roles is in the inflammatory response, but they have a variety of other actions. It was noted that when one of the prostaglandins known as $F_{2\alpha}$ was administered in monkey eyes, a lowering of IOP resulted.[17] Naturally occurring prostaglandin $F_{2\alpha}$ caused pain, headache and conjunctival hyperaemia, therefore the molecule was modified to

Table 10.16	Prostaglandin $F_{2\alpha}$ analogues and their dosages and times of action			
Drug	Commercial product	Onset of lowering of IOP	Time to maximum lowering of IOP	Duration of IOP lowering effect
Bimatoprost	Lumigan® 0.03% (preserved)	4 hours	8 to 12 hours	24 hours
Latanoprost	Xalatan® 0.005% (preserved) Xalacom® (timolol 0.5% with latanoprost 0.005%) (preserved)	3 to 4 hours	8 to 12 hours	24 hours
Travoprost	Travatan® 0.004% (preserved)	2 hours	12 hours	>24 hours

produce a compound with a more favourable adverse effect profile.

Latanoprost and travoprost are prodrugs with good corneal penetration and are converted to the active acid forms. There are different prostanoid (prostaglandin) receptors and latanoprost and travoprost act mainly at the FP receptor. The FP receptor has been located on the ciliary muscle cells of the monkey.[18] It is not known how stimulation of the FP receptor mediates improved uveoscleral outflow, but it is believed that matrix metalloproteinases are involved, which in turn may affect collagen deposition.

Bimatoprost is a synthetic prostamide. The receptors involved in the lowering of intraocular pressure have not yet been positively identified. Pressure lowering is thought to be due to an increase in both trabecular and uveoscleral outflow.

10.8.4 MAIN ADVERSE EFFECTS DUE TO PHARMACOLOGICAL ACTIONS

Ocular adverse effects

Prostaglandins are involved in the inflammatory response and adverse effects are likely to be those associated with this response, although the latanoprost molecule has been modified to limit these effects. Foreign body sensation during the first couple of days of treatment and conjunctival hyperaemia, which is more pronounced initially then subsides as treatment is continued, are both commonly observed.

Prostaglandin analogues may cause an increase in brown pigment of the iris, especially in patients with mixed coloured irides, e.g. blue/brown, green/brown, yellow/brown and gray/brown. This change occurs gradually and may not be noticed for several months or years. It is believed that this colour change is permanent. The brown colour is due to an increase in the pigment melanin which is contained in the stromal melanocytes of the iris. These drugs may also cause darker, longer or thicker eye lashes. Rare cases of macular oedema in aphakic or pseudophakic patients have been reported. There have also been rare reports of iritis/uveitis.

Systemic adverse effects

Systemic adverse effects from topical prostaglandin analogues are uncommon. Rare cases of asthma and exacerbation of the condition have been reported.

10.9 SUMMARY

It can be seen that the mechanisms of action of many of the drugs used in the management of glaucoma are not fully understood. A thorough search of the literature reveals a number of papers that contradict one another regarding the effects of pharmacological agents on aqueous humour dynamics. This may be due to the kind of animal studied and how the results have been extrapolated to man. Animals may have different autonomic innervation or different anatomy to humans.

Measurements of aqueous humour dynamics such as aqueous formation and outflow were usually achieved by indirect methods such as tonography, which is no longer performed, and fluorophotometry, which is a measure of the rate of disappearance of fluorescein from the anterior chamber. Both these methods are subject to errors as the calculations made a number of assumptions that would not hold true today.

The challenge facing ophthalmology today is to devise more appropriate methods that unequivocally establish precise modes of action of drugs to enhance our knowledge and understanding of ocular pharmacology.

References

1. European Glaucoma Society (EGS). Terminology and Guidelines for Glaucoma 2003. Available at: www.eugs.org (accessed 28 September 2005).
2. Breckenridge A. Which beta blocker? BMJ (Clin Res Ed) 1983; 286:1085–1088.
3. Nathanson JA. Human ciliary process adrenergic receptor: pharmacological characterization. Invest Ophthalmol Vis Sci 1981; 21:798–804.
4. Bill A. Effects of norepinephrine, isoproterenol and sympathetic stimulation on aqueous humour dynamics in vervet monkeys. Exp Eye Res 1970; 10:31–46.
5. Ross RA, Drance SM. Effects of topically applied isoproterenol on aqueous dynamics in man. Arch Ophthalmol 1970; 83:39–46.
6. Coakes RL, Brubaker RF. The mechanism of timolol in lowering intraocular pressure in the normal eye. Arch Ophthalmol 1978; 96:2045–2048.
7. Allen RC, Epstein DL. Additive effect of betaxolol and epinephrine in primary open angle glaucoma. Arch Ophthalmol 1986; 104:1178–1184.
8. Thomas JV, Epstein DL. Timolol and epinephrine in primary open angle glaucoma. Transient additive effect. Arch Ophthalmol 1981; 99:91–95.
9. Grierson I, Lee WR, Abraham S. Effects of pilocarpine on the morphology of the human outflow apparatus. Br J Ophthalmol 1978; 62:302–313.
10. Abramson DH, Coleman DJ, Forbes MF. L.A. Pilocarpine. Effect on the anterior chamber and lens thickness. Arch Ophthalmol 1972; 87:615–620.
11. Zimmerman TJ. Pilocarpine. Ophthalmology 1981; 88:85–88.
12. Schenker HI, Yablonski ME, Podos SM, et al. Fluorophotometric study of epinephrine and timolol in human subjects. Arch Ophthalmol 1981; 99:1212–1216.
13. Townsend DJ, Brubacker RF. Immediate effect of epinephrine on aqueous formation in the normal human eye as measured by fluorophotometry. Invest Ophthalmol Vis Sci 1980; 19:256–266.
14. Toris CB, Gleason ML, Camras CB, et al. Effects of brimonidine on aqueous humor dynamics in human eyes. Arch Ophthalmol 1995; 113:1514–1517.
15. Burke J, Padillo E, Shan T, et al. AGN 190342 (UK-14, 304–18) stimulates an imidazoline receptor to lower intraocular pressure (IOP) in conscious monkeys. Invest Ophthalmol Vis Sci 1991; 32 (Suppl):867.
16. Toris CB, Camras CB, Yablonski ME. Effects of PhXA41, a new prostaglandin $F_{2\alpha}$ analog, on aqueous humor dynamics in human eyes. Ophthalmology 1993; 100:1297–1304.
17. Camras CB, Bito LZ. Reduction of intraocular pressure in normal and glaucomatous primate (*Aotus trivirgatus*) eyes by topically applied prostaglandin $F_{2\alpha}$. Curr Eye Res 1981; 1:205–209.
18. Ocklind A, Lake S, Wentzel P, et al. Localization of the prostaglandin $F_{2\alpha}$ receptor in the monkey eye. Invest Ophthalmol Vis Sci 1995; 36 (Suppl):594.

Chapter 11

Medical management of the glaucomas 2

Philip Bloom and Christopher Bentley

11.1 INTRODUCTION

Glaucoma is a leading cause of vision loss (it is estimated to affect 66 million people worldwide, with at least 6.8 million bilaterally blind from the condition[1]) and its treatment has considerable humanitarian, as well as manpower and economic, significance. The only strategy clinically proven so far to slow down the progression of glaucoma is reduction in intraocular pressure (IOP). Historically this has been performed with medication. More recently incisional surgery and laser surgery have also been shown to be effective methods of IOP reduction.

With the evolution of different treatments for glaucoma, the place of medications relative to other treatments such as laser and surgery has therefore changed in recent years. By and large, medical treatments for glaucoma still occupy the first line of most treatment paradigms in modern glaucoma management because of their perceived safety in terms of a risk/benefit analysis. There are, however, some notable exceptions – the management of infantile glaucoma is mainly surgical and closed or narrow angle glaucoma is usually treated initially by laser iridotomy.

11.2 HISTORICAL PERSPECTIVE

Glaucoma may have been recognised as a condition characterised by raised IOP by Arabian writers as long ago as the tenth century, but the first suggestion of medical treatment for the condition was probably made by Sir William Read who reported good results from the administration of 'vegetable decoctions'.[2] Nonetheless there was no effective treatment for this condition until von Graefe introduced his surgical technique for treatment of the acute crisis of closed angle glaucoma in 1856. It was not until the advent of parasympathomimetic topical agents in the late 1870s that a choice was available between medical and surgical treatment modalities.

Physostigmine, a short-acting anticholinesterase agent, was the first agent used for the treatment of glaucoma in 1876 by Lacquer, reputedly on his own eyes.[3] It is derived from the Calabar bean, which grows in west Africa. The alkaloid as the sulphate (eserine) is available in 0.5–1.0% solution and produces prolonged miosis (12–36 hours) although its effect on IOP is less prolonged. Due to the high prevalence of side effects and the advent of newer, more effective, agents, this drug along with a number of other anticholinesterases (demecarium bromide, isoflurophate and echothiophate iodide) is not used now. Another parasympathomimetic that has been in use for over a century is pilocarpine. This was first used for the treatment of glaucoma in 1877 by Weber.[4] This drug is also a naturally occurring alkaloid and is obtained from the leaves of a South American plant, the Jaborandi bush (*Pilocarpus pennatifolius*).

The next group of medications to become available to the ophthalmologist for treatment of glaucoma were the adrenergic agonists. These were first formulated for use as eye drops in glaucoma in the early twentieth century.[5,6] Once initial instability problems were overcome, the drugs gained widespread acceptance, particularly when the prodrug dipivefrine hydrochloride (Propine®) was introduced. This had the advantage of pharmacological inactivity until tissue enzymes hydrolyse it to the active form, so decreasing the systemic side effects. A further step forward was the report by Becker in 1954 that a carbonic anhydrase inhibitor, acetazolamide, lowered IOP in humans.[7] Acetazolamide and other carbonic anhydrase inhibitors (CAIs) are potent systemic medications that lower IOP by reducing the formation of aqueous humour. They inhibit carbonic anhydrase, an enzyme in the ciliary epithelium necessary for the

secretion of aqueous humour. These drugs were found to be extremely effective in reducing IOP in the acute setting and are still widely used.

The introduction of the β-adrenergic agents was a major advance. It was shown in 1967[8] that intravenous propranolol lowered IOP in glaucomatous eyes. Ten years later timolol became available in the maleate form and is the most widely used β-adrenergic agent.[9] A recent advance has been the introduction of once daily dosage regimens for topical β-blockers and of lower drug concentrations. Systemic administration of CAIs has long been acknowledged as an effective way of lowering IOP by reducing aqueous humour production. However oral CAIs are associated with significant systemic side effects, limiting their usefulness in many patients and for long-term therapy. The search for a topically active formulation dates back to the 1950s and finally became available in the mid-1990s in the form of dorzolamide hydrochloride, an agent that is active topically and has mean reductions in IOP comparable to β-blockers.[10] A newer, highly selective α_2-agonist (brimonidine tartrate) that had been shown to reduce IOP in animals and normal humans then became available. It reduces aqueous humour flow and increases outflow facility in normal eyes, in ocular hypertension and open angle glaucoma.[11] Used as a 0.2% solution it has IOP-lowering effects at least comparable to timolol.[12]

The latest chapter in medical management of glaucoma started with the introduction of the 'hypotensive lipid' latanoprost. This prostaglandin $F_{2\alpha}$ analogue was specifically developed for the treatment of glaucoma. It behaves as a selective FP (prostanoid) receptor agonist, its principal mode of action being increased uveoscleral outflow of aqueous.[13] This route is attractive because it is high flow and bypasses the obstructed site of normal drainage. This drug offers additive effects to β-blockade, is mediated via a different route and is without the side effects of miosis and ciliary spasm seen with pilocarpine.

Initially the newer agents were only licensed if first-line drugs such as β-blockers were contraindicated or were ineffective. More recently, many of these agents have been re-licensed as primary therapy, and as a consequence β-blockers have largely been superseded as first-line therapy by the prostaglandin analogues. The most recent advance

Table 11.1 **Relationship between postoperative intraocular pressure (IOP) and progression of visual field loss[16]**

IOP (mmHg)	Percentage with field loss	Follow up (years)	Authors
14.4	6	5	Roth et al 1991[17]
15.0	18	5	Kidd and O'Connor 1985[18]
15.7	10	>4	Kolker 1977[19]
16.0	35	3.5	Werner et al 1977[20]
17.3	35	4	Greve and Dake 1979[21]
18.1	29	5	Rollins and Drance 1981[22]
19.1	58	5	Roth et al 1991[17]

in medical therapy has been the combination of the β-blocker timolol with other agents such as dorzolamide (Cosopt®), latanoprost (Xalacom®), brimonidine (Combigan®), bimatoprost (Ganfort®) and travoprost (DuoTrav®).

11.3 THE PLACE OF MEDICAL TREATMENT FOR GLAUCOMA

The tenet of initial medical therapy has itself also been challenged by some authors. There is evidence that the degree of IOP reduction is less marked using initial glaucoma therapy with medicines than with surgery, and possibly also less effective with medicines than with initial laser treatment.[14] If medical treatment lowers IOP less than other treatments, this suggests that it is less effective than these alternative treatments.

Until recently, the principle that preservation of visual function is linked to the magnitude of IOP reduction in glaucoma patients had not been definitively proved to universal satisfaction.[15] Despite such pessimism there is much evidence, albeit previously circumstantial, of the benefits of IOP reduction in glaucoma. One piece of such evidence is the fact that in patients presenting with glaucoma, the visual field and optic nerve are almost always more affected in the eye with the higher pressure. Moreover, meta-analyses of the literature have long suggested a reasonably close correlation between IOP reduction and the extent of visual field preservation. Table 11.1 shows the results of one such meta-analysis.[16]

Now the results of a number of large, multicentre studies conducted over the last 15 years have been reported,[23,24] these have confirmed the previously anecdotal impression that lower IOP is correlated with preservation of visual field. In one study comparing initial medical and surgical treatment of glaucoma, patients presenting with the mildest visual field defects at diagnosis demonstrated the most severe progressive field loss.[25,26] This apparently paradoxical and counterintuitive finding was interpreted as showing that visual field is lost during the period in which medical treatment is tried unsuccessfully. If this is the case, then the problem may be compounded by the plethora of new pharmaceutical agents currently available or to be introduced in the future. Slavish adherence to a failing medical strategy for glaucoma treatment should obviously be avoided. However, a more recent and much larger study, the Collaborative Initial Glaucoma Treatment Study (CIGTS),[27] demonstrated no difference in visual field survival between patients receiving surgical or medical therapy.

There are of course potential risks and benefits to all methods of IOP reduction. As suggested above, surgery probably lowers IOP more than alternative treatments. This is, however, at the potential risk of complications such as bleb leaks, endophthalmitis, cataract formation, aqueous misdirection, hypotonic maculopathy, suprachoroidal effusion or haemorrhage. Laser treatment is generally held to be safe, but may not be as effective as surgery and may fail relatively suddenly, necessitating continued close observation.

It should be noted that most of the foregoing discussions relate to primary open angle glaucoma (POAG). In the treatment of the secondary glaucomas, it is important also to treat the cause of the increased IOP, which may minimise or abolish the need for glaucoma medications. For example neovascular glaucoma may be treated by panretinal photocoagulation, uveitic glaucoma by topical steroids and silicone oil glaucoma by removal of the silicone oil.

11.4 SIDE EFFECTS OF MEDICAL TREATMENT

Medical treatments themselves are not without drawbacks and side effects, both local and systemic.

11.4.1 LOCAL SIDE EFFECTS

Application of drops may have topical side effects such as burning or stinging due to conjunctival inflammation, ectropion or punctal stenosis due to conjunctival fibrosis, and blurring of vision, miosis, mydriasis or brow ache due to effects on the ciliary muscle. Some drops may also lead to an unpleasant taste, due to nasolacrimal drainage. Some patients tolerate brinzolamide (Azopt®) better than dorzolamide as the former is formulated as a suspension and has a less acidic pH. Local side effects are commonly related to the drug used but may be related to preservative toxicity. A limited number of agents are available in unpreserved unit dose preparations, in order to minimise this problem.

First-generation adrenergic agents were known to cause the deposition of black adrenochrome deposits in the conjunctiva of 20% of patients undergoing chronic therapy.[28] Adrenaline (epinephrine) can be oxidized to adrenochrome (a melanin pigment). More recently it has been discovered that latanoprost may cause irreversible increased pigmentation of the iris, especially in mid-brown irides.[29] Latanoprost may also cause excessive growth and curliness of eyelashes, or periocular pigmentation in a number of individuals. These side effects may be particularly troublesome in patients receiving treatment to one eye only, as they may result in marked asymmetry. Furthermore, there have been reports of uveitis

and cystoid macular oedema in patients using latanoprost, particularly in the presence of aphakia.[30] Dorzolamide is a topical agent that acts by inhibiting the carbonic anhydrase system. Carbonic anhydrase activity maintains the function of the corneal endothelium pump, and so carbonic anhydrase inhibitors may potentiate corneal oedema in those with compromised corneal endothelial function.

Another local side effect of long-term topical medication is that of subconjunctival fibrosis. This is more common with certain agents (such as adrenaline and its precursor drug dipivefrine), and the prevalence rises with increasing duration of therapy and number of agents used.[25,26] This may not be problematical until the patient later comes to surgery due to failure of medical therapy. There may then be an excessively swift and prolonged healing response in the immediate postoperative phase following drainage surgery (such as trabeculectomy) in those patients who have previously used a number of different drops over many years. The scarring caused in this way at the operation site may cause surgery to fail partially or completely.

11.4.2 SYSTEMIC SIDE EFFECTS

Systemic agents such as oral acetazolamide often cause constitutional side effects, including paraesthesia, lethargy, nausea and gastrointestinal disturbances. In addition, there is a degree of systemic absorption from the topical application of all agents via the lacrimal system and nasal mucosa. This gives the potential for systemic side effects from topical agents, which patients may not attribute to their drops unless this has specifically been explained.

Perhaps the most serious systemic side effect of topical medication is that of bronchospasm with topical β-blockers. This potentially fatal side effect[31] is mediated via bronchiolar β-receptors. Less commonly, bronchospasm may also be seen with prostaglandin analogues. Other systemic side effects of β-blockers include cardiovascular effects such as bradycardia (slow pulse) or postural hypotension, and neurological side effects such as nightmares, lethargy and erectile dysfunction. The pulmonary effects may be minimised by the use of the 'cardioselective' agent betaxolol, so called because of its relative affinity for the β_1 (cardiac) over the β_2 (pulmonary) adrenergic receptors.

The use of parasympathetic agents such as pilocarpine may be associated with such side effects as sweating, bradycardia, hypersalivation, bronchospasm and intestinal colic following systemic absorption. Brimonidine can cause dry mouth, and also crosses the blood–brain barrier. For this reason it may cause central nervous system (CNS) effects such as headache, fatigue and drowsiness.[32] In children these effects are particularly marked, and there have been reports of CNS depression.[33] Brimonidine is therefore contraindicated in children.

The side effect profiles of combination drugs are a combination of those of the individual constituents. In blind eyes, pain due to high IOP may be controlled by a combination of topical steroid and cycloplegic drops such as dexamethasone 0.1% four times daily and atropine 1% twice daily.

Notwithstanding the points discussed above, medical glaucoma treatments are regarded overall as safe for the eye, although probably less effective in reducing IOP than surgery. Because of the perceived actuarial advantage in terms of this risk/benefit ratio, initial medical treatment of glaucoma has therefore found wide favour in ophthalmology.

11.4.3 REDUCING SYSTEMIC EFFECTS OF TOPICAL AGENTS

This may be achieved by a variety of means.

- Correct immobilisation of the eyelids to avoid instilling more than the prescribed dose (instillation of multiple doses at intervals of 30 seconds or less increases absorption).
- Digital pressure on the nasolacrimal system at the medial canthus for 3–5 minutes to obstruct drainage to the nose and thus reduce potentially rapid systemic absorption via the nasopharyngeal mucosa.
- Gentle and quiet eyelid closure for 3 minutes after drug instillation.
- Quick blotting away of any excess to reduce the volume of drug administered.
- Use of a local anaesthetic to enhance drug effects by increasing transcorneal absorption and decreasing the dilution effect of tearing caused

by reflex lacrimation from diagnostic or therapeutic drops (used mainly in children).
- Use of semisolid dosage forms such as gels and ointments to alter conjunctival absorption. This decreases passage into the nasolacrimal duct and produces a heightened and prolonged response to a smaller volume of drug than would be required in an aqueous solution.

11.5 ECONOMICS OF GLAUCOMA THERAPY

Cost may also be an issue in the selection of a topical agent to treat glaucoma. The newer agents may be considerably more expensive than older treatments such as pilocarpine.[34] Newer agents may or may not be more effective in lowering IOP than older agents (many comparative studies have yet to be performed), but they certainly have other advantages. It may be argued that it is a matter for debate whether a cost/benefit comparison justifies the widespread use of newer more expensive topical glaucoma medications, at least on current evidence.

In the UK, with a unified prescription charge (£6.65 at the time of writing) to patients within the National Health Service, this cost is borne centrally, but in other countries the cost is directly to the patient. Table 11.2 compares the costs of currently available glaucoma medications in the UK (prices correct at time of going to press). It has been estimated that the total cost associated with each glaucoma patient in the UK is about £12 000 per year. The cost of glaucoma medical therapy must also be balanced against the costs (in human and financial terms) of blindness.[35]

11.6 CURRENT GLAUCOMA TREATMENT STRATEGIES

Prevailing IOP is a balance between aqueous flow in and out of the eye. In reducing IOP, there are three basic medical treatment strategies:

- Reduction of inflow by agents which decrease aqueous secretion, such as β-blockers, carbonic anhydrase inhibitors and α_2-agonists.

Table 11.2   Monthly cost of some selected glaucoma medications in the UK, if used according to manufacturer's specification (drops unless specified)

Drug/strength	Frequency	Cost/Month*
Timolol generic	bd	£1.75 (0.25% 5 ml) £1.69 (0.5% 5 ml)
Betoptic® 0.5%	bd	£2.00 (5 ml)
Levobunolol 0.5%	bd	£2.28 (5 ml)
Pilocarpine	Up to 4 times daily	£2.29 (1% 10 ml) £2.83 (4% 10 ml)
Betoptic® S 0.25%	bd	£2.80 (5 ml)
Betagan® 0.5%	bd	£2.85 (5 ml)
Nyogel® 0.1%	od	£2.85 (5 ml)
Timoptol® 0.25%/0.5%	bd	£3.12 (5 ml)
Trusopt®	tds (mono) vs. bd (dual)	£6.33 (5 ml)
Azopt®	bd (tds if required)	£6.90 (5 ml)
Alphagan®	bd	£8.25 (5 ml)
Timoptol® unit dose	bd	£8.45 (30 × 0.25% 0.2 ml) £9.65 (30 × 0.5% 0.2 ml)
Betagan® unit dose	bd	£9.98 (30 × 0.5% 0.4 ml)
Combigan®	bd	£10.00 (5 ml)
Cosopt®	bd	£10.05 (5 ml)
Travatan®	od (nocte)	£11.06 (2.5 ml)
Iopidine® 0.5%	tds	£11.45 (5 ml)
Lumigan®	od (nocte)	£11.46 (3 ml) £10.89 (3 ml from triple pack)
Diamox® SR	1–2 capsules daily	£11.55 (28 capsule pack)
Xalatan®	od (nocte)	£11.95 (2.5 ml)
Acetazolamide 250 mg	0.25–1 g daily in divided doses	£12.68 (112 tablet pack)
DuoTrav®	od (mane or nocte)	£13.20 (2.5 ml) £12.54 (2.5 ml from triple pack)
Ganfort®	od (mane)	£14.58 (3 ml) £12.53 (3 ml from triple pack)
Xalacom®	od (mane)	£15.07 (2.5 ml)

* Prices correct at time of going to press.
od, once per day; bd, twice daily; tds, three times per day; qds, four times per day; mane, early in the morning; nocte, at night time.

- Reduction of IOP by agents which increase outflow via conventional (trabecular) means, such as pilocarpine.
- Increase in outflow by non-conventional (uveoscleral) drainage routes, such as achieved by prostaglandin (PG) analogues. Some drugs act via more than one mode of action, for example brimonidine is said to have a dual outflow mechanism, with a combined effect on conventional and non-conventional outflow.

Unproven theoretical strategies for treating glaucoma include neuroprotection, the use of topical agents with intrinsic sympathomimetic activity (ISA), and systemic agents such as calcium channel blockers, vasodilators or blood thinning agents.

All agents in clinical usage at the present time are used to reduce IOP, but some of these same agents are also postulated to have other effects on the progression of glaucoma, such as protection of the optic nerve (neuroprotection) and increased blood flow to the optic nerve head. All of these non-IOP effects are as yet unproved. It is further theorised that other new agents with no effect at all on IOP, such as the N-methyl-D-aspartate (NMDA) antagonist memantine, may slow or prevent glaucoma progression by strategies of neural protection or increased vascular perfusion of the optic nerve. Further evidence is obviously needed in this important area, but such evidence is unlikely to be available for some time as these drugs are only just entering clinical trials.

Medications may initially control IOP well, but subsequently become less effective. This reduced effectiveness of a drug with prolonged administration is known as tachyphylaxis. Evidence of this phenomenon is greatest for β-blockers. In this situation a reverse one-eye trial may be performed, and if evidence of tachyphylaxis is found, an alternative treatment may be given. The phenomenon may be drug-specific rather than class specific,[36] so it may be worth trying a different drug of the same class (for example, substituting levobunolol for timolol).

Furthermore, it has been noted that there are non-responders among patients treated for glaucoma with some pharmaceutical agents, and this has been reported recently with latanoprost and dorzolamide.[37,38] In other words, among all patients receiving these treatments, most respond well in terms of IOP reduction, but some not at all. This also means that the figures quoted for the mean IOP reduction of these treatments are skewed downwards. It is likely that many other glaucoma drugs are subject to the same phenomenon, another important reason to assess the response of individual patients to a treatment, and to discontinue the treatment if it does not work.

In any glaucoma treatment, it is important not to lose sight of the needs of the individual patient. Treatments should be tailored to specific needs, responses and side effects. Explanation should be given to patients about the long-term nature of the disease and its treatment, and the possibility of systemic side effects, that may not be otherwise expected, should be stressed.

11.7 MECHANICS OF PRESENT DAY MEDICAL TREATMENTS

Drugs used to treat glaucoma are often considered as either 'first-line', or 'second-line' agents. As the term suggests, the first-line agents are tried first, and second-line agents added or substituted if these do not work. In practice, the first-line agents tend to be those with which there is most clinical experience, for example β-blockers.

This distinction between first-line and second-line treatments is of course artificial, and depends on factors such as length of time on the market, evidence base (which is greater for older drugs), personal preference, side effect profile for the individual and so on. Some drops, however, are not in fact licensed for first-line use in the UK. For example brimonidine (Alphagan®) is recommended for use in patients in whom β-blockers are inappropriate or when β-blockers have failed to control the IOP adequately. In practice this distinction is blurred and it is likely that many of these 'restrictions' will be lifted in time.

Initial medical treatment is almost always with a single drop (monotherapy). If this single agent has little or no effect, then another agent may be substituted. If the effect of a single agent is inadequate, then another agent or agents may be added (dual or multiple therapy). It is interesting to compare relative efficacy of single agent drugs in lowering IOP.[39] Most studies demonstrate a 20–28% reduction in

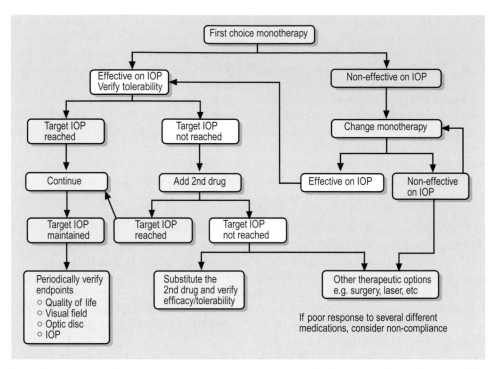

Fig. 11.1   The 2003 European Glaucoma Society treatment algorithm.[43] (Reproduced from European Glaucoma Society, IInd Edition, Chart VIII, with permission from the publisher.)

IOP with topical timolol used as a single hypotensive agent. The effect of latanoprost may be even greater with the mean IOP reduction from baseline ranging from 20% to 36%.[40]

Topical CAIs may be less effective than timolol. In a large double masked trial of 523 glaucoma and ocular hypertensive patients on dorzolamide 2% three times daily versus betaxolol 0.5% twice daily and timolol 0.5% twice daily, the peak pressure reduction at 2 hours post-dose was 23%, 21%, and 25% for dorzolamide, betaxolol, and timolol, respectively.[41] The 8-hour post-dose reductions were 17%, 15%, and 20% respectively, suggesting that dorzolamide is intermediate in efficacy between betaxolol and timolol.

One-eye therapeutic trials, or unilateral trials, involve treatment to one eye only using the other eye as a control. Such an approach permits assessment of the efficacy of individual drugs and discontinuation of ineffective drugs, thus avoiding unnecessary side effects, inconvenience and cost.[42] Caution must be exercised in interpreting the results of one-eye trials, however, as both eyes do not necessarily have similar short and long-term IOP fluctuations. Reverse one-eye trials (one-eye

discontinuation trials), in which a drug is discontinued in only one eye, may also provide useful information by assessing whether a drug is still effective after prolonged use.

In discontinuing any medication, it is important to allow a 'wash-out' period before the effect of the change is finally assessed, as there can be continued effects for some time. The exact duration of this effect varies between drugs from 5 days to 4 weeks, so it is prudent to allow a 1-month washout period. Obviously, new medications should not be started in this time to avoid confusion. Close observation is needed to ensure that on discontinuation of any medication, IOP does not rise to a level that might cause rapid progression of glaucomatous damage.

The mechanics of initiating and amending medical therapies to obtain optimum results for glaucoma treatment have recently been covered in great detail in guidelines from the European Glaucoma Society (EGS).[43] In particular, these guidelines most usefully introduce the concept of 'switching' as opposed to 'adding' medications according to initial effect. Figure 11.1 shows the 2003 EGS treatment algorithm.

11.8 DRUG COMBINATION

The effect of different drugs used together is not necessarily additive. Some medications work synergistically, that is, the overall effect may be as great as or greater than the sum of the individual agents. This tends to be the case for drugs with different mechanisms of action (e.g. β-blockers with pilocarpine). Other drugs work antagonistically, that is the combined action is no better than one or other of the individual effects, and may be worse. This is so when drugs have similar or competing modes of action (e.g. acetazolamide with dorzolamide or pilocarpine with latanoprost). Some of these interactions are theoretically based and some effects are based on clinical evidence, and many practitioners will try various combinations in order to find a 'cocktail' that is effective for an individual patient with acceptable side effects.

In the past, the concept of 'maximum medical treatment' was stressed. In the days when there were a limited number of agents from which to choose, this meant in practical terms that a patient was on most topical treatments available. If topical agents failed to control glaucoma, then an oral CAI was commonly added. In more recent times, this concept has been amended to 'maximum tolerated medical treatment'. This recognises that there is a practical limit to how many drops we can reasonably expect a patient to instil per day, and a limit to patient tolerance with respect to side effects, especially when incremental benefits are ever smaller the more drugs are being used.

Increasingly, treatment of patients with glaucoma focuses not only on clinical effectiveness but also on quality of life issues. Drugs applied once a day are obviously preferred to those used four times a day. Compliance is known to be better with fewer agents prescribed, and with reduced dosage frequency.[44] Those drugs with the fewest topical side effects are preferred, as are those with no systemic side effects. Systemic treatments (such as acetazolamide) are increasingly being abandoned in the treatment of open angle glaucoma for just such reasons, as side effects are common and are potentially dangerous.

Some drugs are combined together in a single formulation, but in the UK there are currently only a limited number of such agents. The first to be introduced was Cosopt®, a combination of timolol 0.5% with dorzolamide 2%. More recently, Xalacom® has been released, a combination of latanoprost with timolol 0.5%. A further combination drug, Combigan®, a combination of brimonidine and timolol 0.5%, was released in the UK in 2005. Most recently Ganfort® (bimatoprost and timolol 0.5%) and DuoTrav® (travoprost and timolol 0.5%) have been released; further combination agents are anticipated. Another example not available in the UK is Timpilo® (available, for example, in Australasia and Canada), a combination of timolol and pilocarpine available in various combination strengths.

The reason there are not more of such combination agents is partly due to formulation issues such as problems with drug stability, and partly because there is little obvious financial benefit to manufacturers in developing these agents. The benefits to patients are obvious, with fewer drops to manage and apply; it is likely that in this way compliance would be improved.

11.9 TARGET PRESSURE

The idea of a 'target pressure' in the treatment of patients with glaucoma has recently been popularised.[45] This recognises the individuality of the needs of each patient in terms of the IOP attained by treatment to try to minimise progression. Patients with more advanced glaucoma benefit from lower target pressure, especially if their life expectancy is greater. Medical treatments may be amended and adjusted by titration against target pressure.

Once a patient's IOP has been stabilised on treatment at an IOP appropriate to the severity of their glaucoma, they should be assessed at regular intervals. Depending on various factors, including disease severity, age, general health and side effects, the frequency of this assessment may be 3–12 monthly. This interval may also be affected by factors such as the need for visual field and optic disc assessment.

The concept of target pressure may also be applied to the treatment of ocular hypertension (OHT). Most ophthalmologists in the UK are prepared to observe patients with OHT, and the results of the recent Ocular Hypertension Treatment Study (OHTS) allow an informed decision about the level of IOP at which it is appropriate to treat any individual patient. Traditionally, treatment for OHT has been instituted with IOPs in the high 20s, or lower if there are any other risk factors such as positive family history, previous venous occlusive disease, aphakia and so on. In addition, it now appears that central corneal thickness and cup/disc ratio are also risk factors, as the OHTS[46] has indicated.

The treatment of normal tension glaucoma (NTG) is more controversial. The only proven strategy for delaying progression of any form of glaucoma is to lower IOP. However, most glaucoma drugs do not lower IOP much, if at all, if the IOP is already in the normal range as in NTG. Latanoprost is an exception, and many clinicians therefore feel that this drug may be of benefit in NTG, although no evidence yet exists to confirm or refute this suggestion. Other strategies proposed to treat NTG include increasing optic nerve head blood flow (for example with betaxolol), the application of neuroprotective agents and surgical intervention.[47]

11.10 NEUROPROTECTION

Neuroprotection is a developing field in medicine. Lowering IOP is an effective neuroprotective strategy in glaucoma, and advances in this area may lead to the development of agents for IOP-independent neuroprotection. These neuroprotective treatments may be given topically, such as brimonidine, which is postulated to have an effect via IOP-dependent and independent means. Alternatively they may be given systemically, the NMDA antagonist memantine, derived from amantadine, shows promise.[48] Calcium channel blockers such as nifedipine are also undergoing evaluation.[49]

Moreover, treatment paradigms are constantly changing with the introduction of new treatments, and it is important to adapt practice to these new advances. New drugs on the horizon at present include ocular hypotensive lipids, similar in action to PGF-2α analogue drugs, NMDA antagonists and calcium channel blockers.

11.11 OCULAR BLOOD FLOW IN GLAUCOMA

It has long been thought that the progression of glaucomatous optic neuropathy may correlate with abnormalities of ocular blood flow (OBF), in particular optic nerve head blood flow. There is some evidence for this, but measurement of OBF is difficult and results open to a number of differing interpretations. Below is given an overview of the subject of OBF in glaucoma, and effects of treatment.

Patients with raised IOP due to POAG have reduced ophthalmic artery blood flow velocity[50,51] and reduction in macular blood cell velocity proportional to disease severity.[52] In NTG, patients have been shown to have an age-related increase in ophthalmic artery resistance.[53] One study has found that patients with glaucoma (both POAG and NTG) have reduced blood flow velocity in the optic nerve head capillaries as measured by Laser Doppler Velocimetry (LDV), and increased aggregability of red blood cells.[54]

There is significantly lower pulsatile ocular blood flow (POBF) in patients with POAG than in those with OHT,[55] and lower POBF in patients with NTG than normals.[56] The normal physiological POBF reduction in the supine posture[57] may result in tissue hypoxia in subjects with, or at risk of developing, glaucoma or conditions of vascular insufficiency; this may explain the common observation that vascular occlusions commonly occur at night. Furthermore, nocturnal arterial hypotension, in the presence of other vascular risk factors, also plays a role in the pathogenesis of these conditions by reducing the blood supply of the optic nerve head to below a critical level.[58] The characteristic patterns of visual field loss in POAG and NTG follow the horizontal midline, reflecting the altitudinal blood supply to the retina and retrolaminar optic nerve head, and acute hypovolaemic shock is a cause of non-progressive altitudinal visual field defects.

Many studies have examined the effect of different autonomic agents upon the ocular circulation, but results are difficult to interpret because of the combined effects of these drugs on blood flow, IOP and systemic blood pressure. For example, instillation of timolol reduces IOP causing increased perfusion pressure; the resulting retinal arteriolar vasoconstriction[59] may therefore be due to a compensatory autoregulation effect.

Pilocarpine has no direct effect on POBF.[60] Studies of POBF following treatment with β-blockers have been inconclusive. One study found that POBF was not altered by timolol treatment,[60] but another found that levobunolol had a similar effect in normal and glaucoma patients, decreasing IOP by about 30% and increasing POBF by about 12%.[61] In the same study the ocular pulse volume amplitude increased with levobunolol by 42% in normal eyes but was unchanged in glaucomatous eyes.[62] POBF has been found to decrease in timolol-treated eyes over 1 year, but is stable in betaxolol-treated eyes.[62]

LDV studies have demonstrated that carteolol (a β-blocker with 'intrinsic sympathomimetic activity'), has no effect on retinal blood flow,[63] but have shown timolol to increase retinal blood flow by about 12%[64,65] and betaxolol by 15%.[66] The systemic CAI acetazolamide reduces IOP and has been shown by LDV to cause vasodilatation and to increase retinal blood flow, an effect that may be mediated via local alterations of the partial pressure of carbon dioxide. It has been shown using colour Doppler imaging that timolol instilled in one eye causes a reduction in the mean resistive index of both that and the fellow eye,[67] which has been interpreted as representing a reduction in peripheral vascular resistance. Further research is needed to determine the effect on OBF of newer ocular hypotensive agents, such as α-agonists (e.g. apraclonidine and brimonidine), topical CAIs (e.g. dorzolamide), prostaglandins (e.g. the PGF-2 ester latanoprost) and various dopaminergic agents.

Following surgical treatment of POAG, central retinal artery and posterior ciliary artery flow velocities increase, probably because IOP has decreased.[68] Despite the evidence outlined above concerning the effects of medical treatments on OBF, currently only betaxolol (Betoptic®) is listed as maintaining or increasing ocular blood flow/perfusion.[69] At the present time the clinical role of blood flow measurements in glaucoma management (and the relevance of changes noted with drug treatments) is unclear and these techniques remain research tools. It is anticipated that with further investigation and future technological improvements, these methods of examination will be incorporated into routine clinical practice.

11.12 CONCLUSION

There is evidence as to the benefit of medical treatment of glaucoma. Strategies for medical treatment currently centre upon lowering IOP, and with the increasing numbers of new pharmaceutical agents there are ever more ways of achieving IOP reduction. It is important, however, not to lose sight of the patient as an individual, and treatment must be tailored to particular circumstances and needs.

It is important also to know when medicines are not achieving the targets of treatment so that alternative treatments, be they laser or surgical, may be planned. Slavish adherence to a failing medical strategy for glaucoma treatment should obviously be avoided, as by this means visual function may be adversely affected in the long term.

APPENDIX 1

PHARMACOPOEIA OF SOME OF THE MOST COMMONLY USED GLAUCOMA MEDICATIONS AVAILABLE IN THE UK (TO BE USED IN CONJUNCTION WITH MANUFACTURERS' DATA SHEETS)

Prostaglandin analogues/prostamide

These drugs include prostaglandin PGF-2α analogues and prostamide drugs, the latter said to act via a different receptor.[70] They lower IOP by enhancing uveoscleral outflow, although the exact mechanism underlying this remains unclear; one hypothesis is that prostaglandins may stimulate collagenase and other metalloproteinases to degrade the extracellular matrix between ciliary muscle bundles.[71] These drugs are now licensed for first-line use, and are also used as adjunctive treatments. They are contraindicated in pregnancy and lactation.

Side effects include: iris hyperpigmentation, transient irritation and hyperaemia, allergic conjunctivitis, and corneal punctate epithelial erosions.

- Drug name
- Dosage
- Proprietary name (manufacturer)
- Excipients include
- Different forms

Bimatoprost (300 μg/ml)
One drop daily (preferably in the evening)
Lumigan® (Allergan)
Benzalkonium chloride
Ganfort® (with timolol)

- Drug name
- Dosage
- Proprietary name (manufacturer)
- Excipients include
- Different forms

Latanoprost (50 μg/ml)
One drop daily (preferably in the evening)
Xalatan® (Pfizer)
Benzalkonium chloride
Xalacom® (with timolol)

- Drug name
- Dosage
- Proprietary name (manufacturer)
- Excipients include
- Different forms

Travoprost (40 μg/ml)
One drop daily (preferably in the evening)
Travatan® (Alcon)
Benzalkonium chloride
DuoTrav® (with timolol)

β-blockers

These have traditionally formed the mainstay of medical management, and are now often also used as adjunctive treatments; timolol is used in a number of fixed combination therapies. β-blockers have side effects that limit their usefulness due to systemic absorption via the nasolacrimal mucosa (i.e. bypassing first pass metabolism) particularly in patients with chronic obstructive airways disease or asthma and patients with cardiac conduction defects.[72]

These medications lower IOP by reducing the rate of aqueous humour formation and have no effect on pupil size, accommodation, or outflow facility.[73,74] They may be cardioselective/non-selective, and dosage is usually twice daily. Contraindications include: heart block, bradycardia, uncompensated cardiac failure, asthma, and chronic obstructive pulmonary disease.

- Drug name
- Dosage
- Proprietary name (manufacturer)
- Excipients include
- Different forms

Betaxolol hydrochloride (0.5%)
One drop twice a day
Betoptic® (Alcon)
Benzalkonium chloride, EDTA
Betoptic® S 0.25% (ophthalmic suspension)

- Drug name
- Dosage

Carteolol hydrochloride (1%)
One drop twice a day

- Proprietary name (manufacturer)   Teoptic® (Novartis)
- Excipients include   Benzalkonium chloride
- Different forms   2%

- Drug name   **Levobunolol hydrochloride** (0.5%)
- Dosage   One drop once or twice a day
- Proprietary name (manufacturer)   Betagan® (Allergan)
- Excipients include   Benzalkonium chloride, EDTA
- Different forms   Unit dose (preservative free)

- Drug name   **Metipranolol** (0.1%)
- Dosage   1 drop twice a day
- Proprietary name   Metipranolol Minims®
- Different forms   0.3%

- Drug name   **Timolol maleate** (0.25%)
- Dosage   One drop twice a day (Timoptol®-LA and Nyogel® once a day)
- Proprietary name (manufacturers)   Timoptol® (MSD), Timoptol®-LA (MSD), Nyogel® (Novartis)
- Excipients include   Benzalkonium chloride
- Different forms   0.5%, Nyogel® 0.1% eye gel, Cosopt® (with dorzolamide), Xalacom® (with latanoprost), Timoptol® unit dose eye drops (preservative free) Combigan® (with Brimonidine), Ganfort® (with Bimatoprost), DuoTrav® (with Travoprost)

Carbonic anhydrase inhibitors

As the name implies, CAIs inhibit carbonic anhydrase, thus reducing the bicarbonate in aqueous humour and the water secreted with it, resulting in decreased aqueous volume and lowered IOP.

When used systemically as acetazolamide, the dosage is usually 250–1000 mg/day. Side effects include electrolyte disturbances, development of renal stones,[75] paraesthesia, initial diuresis, polyuria, metallic taste (probably due to the inhibition of carbonic anhydrase in taste buds), nausea, loss of appetite, depression and general malaise. Contraindications include hypokalaemia, hyponatraemia, hyperchloraemic acidosis, severe hepatic impairment, renal impairment and sulphonamide hypersensitivity.

Topical CAIs are licensed for adjunctive use or if first-line drugs are ineffective or contraindicated. Side effects of topical CAIs include bitter taste, burning, stinging and itching of the eye, blurred vision and tearing. Contraindications include corneal failure, as CAIs inhibit the corneal endothelial cell pump, severe renal impairment, hyperchloraemic acidosis, pregnancy and lactation. A fixed combination of dorzolamide and timolol (Cosopt®) is available.

- Drug name   **Brinzolamide** (10 mg/ml)
- Dosage   One drop twice daily, increasing to three times daily if necessary
- Proprietary name (manufacturer)   Azopt® (Alcon)
- Excipients include   Benzalkonium chloride, EDTA
- Different forms   None

- Drug name   **Dorzolamide hydrochloride** (2%)
- Dosage   One drop three times a day as monotherapy or twice for adjunctive therapy
- Proprietary name (manufacturer)   Trusopt® (MSD)
- Excipients include   Benzalkonium chloride
- Different forms   Cosopt® (with timolol)

Adrenergic agonists

Adrenergic agents are thought to have a dual mechanism of action, reducing aqueous inflow and increasing outflow. Non-selective adrenergic agents are contraindicated in angle-closure in the absence of a patent peripheral iridotomy. Side effects include ocular hyperaemia, conjunctival follicles, stinging, pruritis, oedema, local allergic reactions, dry mouth, headache, fatigue and drowsiness.

Special precautions should be taken in the presence of severe cardiovascular disease, depression, cerebral or coronary insufficiency, Raynaud's syndrome, orthostatic hypotension, renal or hepatic impairment. Contraindications include use in children, pregnancy and lactation; these drugs may also interact with monoamine oxidase inhibitors (MAOIs), antidepressants affecting noradrenergic transmission, CNS depressants, antihypertensives, cardiac glycosides, sympathomimetic agonists or antagonists.

Apraclonidine is often used as the 1% unit dose preparation for very short-term adjunctive use to prevent pressure spikes after anterior segment laser, and instillation is effective either before or after these procedures.[76] Apraclonidine 0.5% may also be used for short-term adjunctive use. Brimonidine is used as an adjunctive treatment or for those for whom first-line treatments are ineffective or contraindicated. A fixed combination of brimonidine and timolol (Combigan®) is available.

- Drug name   **Apraclonidine hydrochloride** (0.5%)
- Dosage   One drop three times daily, usually for a maximum of 1 month
- Proprietary name (manufacturer)   Iopidine® (Alcon)
- Excipients include   Benzalkonium chloride, EDTA
- Different forms   Iopidine® 1% unit dose (preservative free)

- Drug name   **Brimonidine tartrate** (0.2%)
- Dosage   One drop twice daily
- Proprietary name (manufacturer)   Alphagan® (Allergan)
- Excipients include   Benzalkonium chloride
- Different forms   Combigan® (with timolol)

Miotics/parasympathomimetics

The only such drug still in common use in the UK is pilocarpine, which acts by facilitating trabecular meshwork outflow.[77] Pilocarpine is commonly commercially available in strengths of 0.5–4% (a few suppliers produce greater strengths), and is usually administered four times per day; this frequency may hinder patient compliance. Local side effects include headache, brow ache and blurred vision. Systemic parasympathomimetic side effects may also occur, such as sweating, bradycardia, intestinal colic, hypersalivation and bronchospasm (asthma).

Pilocarpine is contraindicated in conditions where pupillary constriction is undesirable, such as acute inflammation of the anterior segment, and may cause reduced vision in the presence of cataract. In the past, a sustained slow-release preparation of pilocarpine (Ocusert Pilo®) was of use in conditions such as pigment dispersion syndrome. This preparation has now been discontinued, but a long-acting gel (Pilogel®) may be of help in similar clinical scenarios.

- Drug name   **Pilocarpine hydrochloride** (0.5–4%)
- Dosage   One drop, four times a day
- Different forms   Pilogel® – 4% ophthalmic gel; Minims® (pilocarpine nitrate 1%, 2% and 4% preservative free)

Older glaucoma drugs

These medications include adrenaline and its analogues or prodrugs (e.g. dipivefrine and guanethidine), and older miotics such as carbachol; they are now rarely if ever used in the UK. Local side effects were common with these medications,[78] and included severe smarting and ocular redness. It is now known that the inflammatory effects on the conjunctiva may adversely affect the outcomes of future filtration surgery[79] after prior treatment with these agents.

References

1. Quigley HA. Number of people with glaucoma worldwide. Br J Ophthalmol 1996; 80:389–93.

2. Duke-Elder S, ed. System of Ophthalmology. St. Louis: Mosby; 1969; Vol XI:381.

3. Laqueur L. Neue therapeutische Indikation für Physostigmine. Centralbl med Wissensch 1876; 14:421.

4. Weber A. Die Ursache des Glaukoms. von Graefe's Arch Ophthalmol 1877; 23:1.

5. Knapp A. The action of adrenalin on the glaucomatous eye. Arch Ophthalmol 1921; 50:556.

6. Gifford SR. Some modern preparations used in the treatment of glaucoma. Arch Ophthalmol 1928; 57:612.

7. Becker B. Decrease in intraocular pressure in man by a carbonic anhydrase inhibitor, Diamox: A preliminary report. Am J Ophthalmol 1954; 37:13.

8. Phillips CI, Howitt G, Rowlands DL. Propranolol as an ocular hypotensive agent. Br J Ophthalmol 1967; 96:2045.

9. Zimmerman TJ, Kaufman HE. Timolol: A beta adrenergic blocking agent for the treatment of glaucoma. Arch Ophthalmol 1977; 95:601.

10. Strahlman E, Tipping R, Vogel R, et al. A double masked, randomised 1-year study comparing Dorzolamide (Trusopt), timolol, and betaxolol. Arch Ophthalmol 1995; 113.1009–1016.

11. Walters TR. Development and use of brimonidine in treating acute and chronic elevations of intraocular pressure: a review of safety, efficacy, dose response, and dosing studies. Surv Ophthalmol 1996; 41(Suppl 1): S19–S26.

12. Schuman JS. Clinical experience with brimonidine 0.2% and timolol 0.5% in glaucoma and ocular hypertension. Surv Ophthalmol 1996; 41(Suppl 1): S27–S37.

13. Sternschantz J, Selén G, Sjöquist B, et al. Preclinical pharmacology of Latanoprost, a phenylsubstituted $PGF_{2\alpha}$ analogue. Vol 23. In: Samuelsson B, ed. Advances in Prostaglandin, Thromboxane and Leukotriene Research. New York: Raven Press; 1995:513–518.

14. Migdal C, Gregory W, Hitchings R. Long term functional outcome after early surgery compared with laser and medicine in open angle glaucoma. Ophthalmology 1994; 101:1651–1656.

15. Smith R. Glaucoma: is there light at the end of the tunnel? Br J Ophthalmol 1990; 74:1–2.

16. Palmberg P. How clinical trials are changing our thinking about target pressures. Curr Opin Ophthalmol 2002; 13:85–88.

17. Roth SM, Spaeth GL, Starita RJ, et al. The effects of postoperative corticosteroids on trabeculectomy and the clinical course of glaucoma: five-year follow-up study. Ophthalmic Surg 1991; 22:724–729.

18. Kidd MN, O'Connor M. Progression of field loss after trabeculectomy: a five-year follow-up. Br J Ophthalmol 1985; 69:827–831.

19. Kolker AE. Visual prognosis in advanced glaucoma: A comparison of medical and surgical therapy for retention of vision in 101 eyes with advanced glaucoma. Trans Am Ophthalmol Soc 1977; 75:539–555.

20. Werner EB, Drance SM, Schultzer M. Trabeculectomy and progression of glaucomatous visual field loss. Arch Ophthalmol 1977; 95:1374–1377.

21. Greve EL, Dake CL. Four-year follow-up of a glaucoma operation. Int Ophthalmol 1979; 1:139–145.

22. Rollins DF, Drance SM. Five year follow-up of trabeculectomy in the management of chronic open angle glaucoma. New Orleans Acad Ophthalmol 1981; 295–300.

23. Nouri-Mahdavi K, Hoffman D, Coleman AL, et al. Advanced Glaucoma Intervention Study. Predictive factors for glaucomatous visual field progression in the Advanced Glaucoma Intervention Study. Ophthalmology 2004; 111:1627–1635.

24. Leske MC, Heijl A, Hussein M, et al. Early Manifest Glaucoma Trial Group. Factors for glaucoma progression and the effect of treatment: the Early Manifest Glaucoma Trial. Arch Ophthalmol 2003; 121:48–56.

25. Jay JL. Rational choice of therapy in primary open angle glaucoma. Eye 1992; 6:243–247.

26. Jay JL, Allan D. The benefit of early trabeculectomy versus conventional management in primary open angle glaucoma relative to severity of disease. Eye 1989; 3:528–535.

27. Musch DC, Lichter PR, Guire KE, et al. CIGTS Investigators: The Collaborative Initial Glaucoma Treatment Study (CIGTS): Study design, methods, and baseline characteristics of enrolled patients. Ophthalmology 1999; 106:653–662.

28. Corwin ME, Spencer WH. Conjunctival melanin depositions. Arch Ophthalmol 1963; 69:317.

29. Watson PG, Stjernschantz J. UK Latanoprost Study Group: Intraocular pressure (IOP) reducing effect and side-effects of latanoprost and timolol: a six-month double-masked comparison. Ophthalmology 1994; 101(suppl):80.

30. Warwar RE, Bullock JD, Ballal D. Cystoid macular edema and anterior uveitis associated with latanoprost use. Ophthalmology 1998; 105:263–268.

31. Van Buskirk EM, Fraunfelder FT. Ocular beta blockers and systemic side effects. Am J Ophthalmol 1994; 98:623–624.

32. Schuman JS, Horwitz B, Choplin NT, et al. A 1-year study of brimonidine twice daily in glaucoma and ocular hypertension. A controlled, randomised, multicenter clinical trial. Arch Ophthalmol 1997; 115:847–852.

33. Carlsen JO, Zabriskie NA, Kwon YH, et al. Apparent central nervous system depression in infants after the use of topical brimonidine. Am J Ophthalmol 1999; 128:255–256.

34. British National Formulary 51. London: British Medical Association and The Royal Pharmaceutical Society of Great Britain; 2006.

35. The Costs of Blindness Report. Reading, Berkshire: Guide Dogs for the Blind Association, July 2003.

36. Kriegelstein GK, Sold-Darseff J, Leydhecker W. The intraocular pressure response of glaucomatous eyes to topically applied bupranolol. A pilot study. Graefe's Arch Clin Exp Ophthalmol 1977; 202:81–86.

37. Yang CB, Freedman SF, Myers JS, et al. Use of latanoprost in the treatment of glaucoma associated with Sturge-Weber syndrome. Am J Ophthalmol 1998; 126:600–602.

38. Detry-Morel M, De-Hoste F. Treatment of glaucoma with carbonic anhydrase inhibitors in eyewash: medium term retrospective experience with dorzolamide. Bull Soc Belge Ophtalmol 1997; 267:157–166.

39. Stewart RH, Kimbrough RL, Ward RL. Betaxold vs timolol. A six-month double-blind comparison. Arch Ophthalmol 1986; 104(1):46–48.

40. Alm A, Camras CB, Watson PG. Phase III latanoprost studies in Scandinavia, the United Kingdom and the United States. Surv Ophthalmol 1997; 41: S105–S110.

41. Strahlman E, Tipping R, Vogel R. A double-masked, randomized 1-year study comparing dorzolamide (Trusopt), timolol and betaxolol. International Dorzolamide Study Group. Arch Ophthalmol 1995; 113(8):1009–1016.

42. Wandel T, Charap AD, Lewis RA, et al. Glaucoma treatment with once daily levobunolol. Am J Ophthalmol 1986; 101:298–304.

43. European Glaucoma Society. Terminology and Guidelines for Glaucoma, IInd Edition. Savona, Italy: DOGMA Srl; 2003.

44. Norell SE, Granstrom PA. Self-medication with pilocarpine among outpatients in a glaucoma clinic. Br J Ophthalmol 1980; 64:137.

45. Anderson DR. Glaucoma: The damage caused by pressure. XLVI Edward Jackson Memorial Lecture. Am J Ophthalmol 1989; 108:485.

46. Gordon MO, Beiser JA, Brandt JD, et al. Ocular Hypertension Treatment Study Group. The Ocular Hypertension Treatment Study. Baseline factors that predict the onset of primary open angle glaucoma. Arch Ophthalmol 2002; 120:714–720.

47. Anonymous. Comparison of glaucomatous progression between untreated patients with normal-tension glaucoma and patients with therapeutically reduced intraocular pressures. Collaborative Normal-Tension Glaucoma Study Group. Am J Ophthalmol 1998; 126:487–497.

48. Chen HSV, Pelligrini JW, Aggarwal SK, et al. Open channel block of N-methyl-D-aspartate (NMDA) responses by memantine: therapeutic advantage against NMDA receptor-mediated neurotoxicity. J Neurosci 1992;12:4427–4436.

49. Netland P, Chaturvedi N, Dreyer EB. Calcium channel blockers in the management of low-tension and open-angle glaucoma. Am J Ophthalmol 1993; 115:608.

50. Rojanapongpun P, Drance SM, Morrison BJ. Ophthalmic artery flow velocity in glaucomatous and normal subjects. Br J Ophthalmol 1993; 77:25–29.

51. Michelson G, Groh MJ, Groh ME, et al. Advanced primary open-angle glaucoma is associated with decreased ophthalmic artery blood-flow velocity. German J Ophthalmol 1995; 4:21–24.

52. Sponsel WE, DePaul KL, Kaufman PL. Correlation of visual function and retinal leukocyte velocity in glaucoma. Am J Ophthalmol 1990; 109:49–54.

53. Butt Z, McKillop G, O'Brien C, et al. Measurement of ocular blood flow velocity using colour Doppler imaging in low tension glaucoma. Eye 1995; 9(Pt 1):29–33.

54. Hamard P, Hamard H, Dufaux J, et al. Optic nerve head blood flow using a laser Doppler velocimeter and haemorheology in primary open angle glaucoma and normal pressure glaucoma. Br J Ophthalmol 1994; 78:449–453.

55. Trew DR, Smith SE. Postural studies in pulsatile ocular blood flow: II. Chronic open angle glaucoma. Br J Ophthalmol 1991; 75:71–75

56. James CB, Smith SE. Pulsatile ocular blood flow in patients with low tension glaucoma. Br J Ophthalmol 1991; 75:466–470.

57. Trew DR, Smith SE. Postural studies in pulsatile ocular blood flow: I. Ocular hypertension and normotension. Br J Ophthalmol 1991; 75:66–70.

58. Hayreh SS, Zimmerman MB, Podhajsky P, et al. Nocturnal arterial hypotension and its role in optic nerve head and ocular ischemic disorders. Am J Ophthalmol 1994; 117:603–624.

59. Martin XD, Rabineau PA. Vasoconstrictive effect of topical timolol on human retinal arteries. Graefes Arch Clin Exp Ophthalmol 1989; 227:526–530.

60. Claridge KG. The effect of topical pilocarpine on pulsatile ocular blood flow. Eye 1993; 7:507–510.

61. Bosem ME, Lusky M, Weinreb RN. Short-term effects of levobunolol on ocular pulsatile flow. Am J Ophthalmol 1992; 114:280–286.

62. Carenini AB, Sibour G, Boles Carenini B. Differences in the longterm effect of timolol and betaxolol on the pulsatile ocular blood flow. Surv Ophthalmol 1994; 38: S118–S124.

63. Grunwald JE, Delehanty J. Effect of topical carteolol on the normal human retinal circulation. Invest Ophthalmol Vis Sci 1992; 33:1853–1856.

64. Grunwald JE. Effect of topical timolol on the human retinal circulation. Invest Ophthalmol Vis Sci 1986; 27:1713–1719.

65. Grunwald JE. Topical timolol and the human retinal circulation. Surv Ophthalmol 1989; 33:415–416.

66. Gupta A, Chen HC, Rassam SM, et al. Effect of betaxolol on the retinal circulation in eyes with ocular hypertension: a pilot study. Eye 1994; 8:668–671.

67. Baxter GM, Williamson TH, McKillop G, et al. Color Doppler ultrasound of orbital and optic nerve blood flow: effects of posture and timolol 0.5%. Invest Ophthalmol Vis Sci 1992; 33:604–610.

68. Trible JR, Sergott RC, Spaeth GL, et al. Trabeculectomy is associated with retrobulbar hemodynamic changes. A colour Doppler analysis. Ophthalmology 1994; 101:340–351.

69. ABPI Compendium of Data Sheets and Summaries of Product Characteristics 1998. London: Datapharm Publications; 20–21.

70. Woodward DF, Krauss AH, Chen J, et al. The pharmacology of bimatoprost (Lumigan). Surv Ophthalmol 2001; 45(Suppl 4): 337–345.

71. Tamm E, Rittig M, Lutjen-Drecoll E. Electromikroskopische and immunohistochemische untersuchungen zur augendrucksenkender wirkung von prostaglandin F2a. Fortschr Ophthalmol 1990; 87:623.

72. Everitt DE, Avorn J. Systemic effects of medications used to treat glaucoma. Ann Intern Med 1990; 112:120–125.

73. Zimmerman TJ, Harbin R, Pett M, et al. Timolol: facility of outflow. Invest Ophthalmol 1977; 16:623.

74. Zimmerman TJ, Kass MA, Yablonski ME, et al. Timolol maleate: Efficacy and safety. Arch Ophthalmol 1979; 97:656.

75. Charron RG, Feldman F. Acetazolamide therapy with renal complications. Can J Ophthalmol 1974; 9:282.

76. Hurvitz LM, Kaufman PL, Robin AL, et al. New developments in the drug treatment of glaucoma. Drugs 1991; 41:514–532.

77. Kaufman PL, Barany EH. Loss of acute pilocarpine effect on outflow facility following surgical disinsertion and retrodisplacement of the ciliary muscle from the scleral spur in the cynomolgus monkey. Invest Ophthalmol 1976; 15:793.

78. Broadway DC, Grierson I, O'Brien C, et al. Adverse effects of topical antiglaucoma medication. I. The conjunctival cell profile. Arch Ophthalmol 1994; 112:1437–1445.

79. Broadway DC, Grierson I, O'Brien C, et al. Adverse effects of topical antiglaucoma medication. II. The outcome of filtration surgery. Arch Ophthalmol 1994; 112:1446–1454.

Chapter 12

Laser and surgical treatment of glaucoma

Mark R Wilkins, Peter Shah and Peng T Khaw

TREATMENT OPTIONS FOR OPEN ANGLE GLAUCOMA

Medical treatment options for open angle glaucoma have been discussed in the two preceding chapters. This chapter will discuss laser (argon laser trabeculoplasty (ATL)) and surgical (trabeculectomy) treatment.

REASONS FOR CHOOSING LASERS OR SURGERY

- Medical treatment is not lowering intraocular pressure (IOP) sufficiently.
- Patient is experiencing adverse effects from medical treatment (see Chapters 10 and 11).
- Patient is not complying with medical treatment.
- Medical treatment cannot be expected to control pressure – for example in an acute attack of angle closure glaucoma.

12.1 ARGON LASER TRABECULOPLASTY

ALT is used in the treatment of open angle glaucoma (including pseudoexfoliation, pigment dispersion syndrome and secondary open angle glaucoma). The laser is not used to make a hole or holes into Schlemm's canal; instead mild blanching laser burns are applied to the trabecular meshwork (TM). This causes trabecular cells in the anterior TM to divide, which stimulates new trabecular cells to migrate over the TM. The result is remodelling of the extracellular matrix stimulated by the migrating cells. In primary open angle glaucoma (POAG) the main resistance to aqueous outflow comes from the trabecular juxtacanalicular matrix. ALT causes remodelling of the matrix leading to reduced resistance to outflow.

The ALT technique is as follows and is performed using a slit-lamp mounted argon laser:

- Apraclonidine drops are given before treatment (and after treatment) to prevent pressure spikes. (Immediately following the procedure there may be a rise of 10–20 mmHg in the IOP, and apraclonidine drops are routinely given to help prevent this occurring.)
- Pilocarpine drops may also be given to improve the view of the angle.
- Local anaesthetic drops are instilled and a gonioscopy lens applied.
- The power of the laser is altered so the TM just whitens after each burn.
- 50 burns are applied over 180° of pigmented TM – nasal or temporal half.
- The patient is given a short course of steroid drops.
- IOP is checked 4–6 weeks later.

12.1.1 OUTCOMES OF ALT

The procedure achieves a 50% success rate at 5 years after surgery.[1] The IOP-lowering effect can wear off at any time following treatment. ALT rarely removes the need for medical therapy, so ALT is used as an additional treatment to drops. Therefore, the ALT procedure prolongs the patient's exposure to anti-glaucoma medication

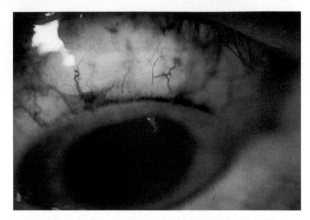

Fig. 12.1   A drainage bleb seen about 1 week after a trabeculectomy. Through the semitransparent conjunctiva can be seen the partial thickness scleral flap in position. The flap is held in position by two sutures which are also visible.

and may thus compromise future filtration surgery. There is a chance of further field loss as the effect of the laser treatment wears off. If this occurs the procedure can be repeated as required, although the reduction in IOP is usually less than after the first treatment. Other complications of ALT include iritis, peripheral synechiae and haemorrhage.

12.2 TRABECULECTOMY ('DRAINAGE' OR 'FILTRATION' SURGERY)

Trabeculectomy is the commonest form of glaucoma surgery in the UK. Its name is a misnomer, because the mechanism of action is not linked to removal of the TM. Instead, a channel/fistula is made through the sclera/limbus from the anterior chamber to the subconjunctival space. Aqueous passes through the fistula in the sclera and collects under the conjunctiva as a bleb (see Fig. 12.1). Aqueous is absorbed by capillaries and lymphatics in the conjunctiva or evaporates across the conjunctiva. The path through the sclera is not a direct hole; it is guarded by a scleral flap. This offers resistance to the flow of aqueous out of the eye preventing hypotony (low IOP) especially in the early postoperative period.

12.2.1 TRABECULECTOMY TECHNIQUE

The operation can be performed under local or general anaesthesia. The globe is positioned in downgaze using a traction suture passing through the stroma of the peripheral cornea at the 12 o'clock position where the operation is performed. The conjunctiva is dissected away from the sclera. A partial-thickness flap is cut in the outer sclera and peeled forwards. A full thickness hole is made in the underlying sclera—a sclerostomy. A special punch is sometimes used. The peripheral iris is pulled through the sclerostomy and a small hole is cut in it—a peripheral iridectomy. The scleral flap is returned to its original position and loosely sutured to produce a guarded sclerostomy. Special releasable/adjustable sutures which are more tightly tied initially are also used. The conjunctiva is replaced and sutured.

Aqueous can now drain from the anterior chamber through the sclerostomy, pass around the edges of the scleral flap and collect under the conjunctiva where it forms a bleb.

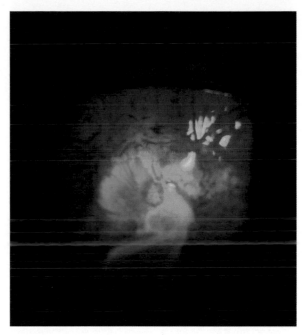

Fig. 12.2 A conjunctival wound leak shown using fluorescein. Aqueous pouring through the conjunctiva dilutes the fluorescein.

12.2.2 EARLY COMPLICATIONS OF TRABECULECTOMY

- Endophthalmitis. This is a devastating infection of the globe which may occur within the first few weeks following any intraocular surgery.
- Uveitis.
- Hyphaema. This may resolve over the first week or two following surgery.
- Under-drainage of aqueous may occur. The scleral flap sutures may be too tight, in which case one or more of the sutures holding down the scleral flap can be released. If regular sutures were used then the argon laser can be used to produce suture lysis. If releasable sutures were used, massaging the eyeball can loosen them or the sutures can be pulled using very fine forceps. Blood or fibrin may also obstruct the sclerostomy. This produces raised IOP and a shallow anterior chamber.
- Over-drainage of aqueous may occur. This may be because the scleral flap is too loose, and this lack of resistance from the flap leads to excessive outflow of aqueous from the eye. Alternatively, there may be conjunctival wound leak, with the result that aqueous is unable to collect in a bleb (Fig. 12.2). In either case this produces low IOP and a shallow anterior chamber, choroidal effusions, macular oedema and choroidal folds. If the anterior chamber is shallow enough to produce lenticulo-corneal touch, then a cataract usually develops. Releasable sutures have been introduced in an effort to prevent hypotony after surgery, especially if antimetabolites (see section 12.2.5) have been used. With this approach, the scleral flap sutures can be tied tight. If IOP is too high in the days and weeks following surgery, the eye can be massaged to loosen the suture or the suture can be removed completely if the pressure remains too high.
- Reduced visual acuity. On average, patients will lose a few letters of acuity. If hypotony occurs, loss of acuity may be the result of macular oedema.

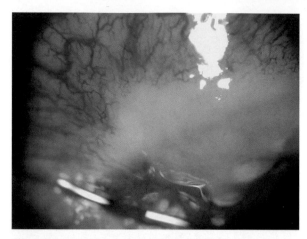

Fig. 12.3 Blebitis – a localised bleb infection.

12.2.3 LATER COMPLICATIONS OF TRABECULECTOMY

- Cataract is common. Of the patients who underwent trabeculectomy as part of the Collaborative Normal-Tension Glaucoma Study 48% developed cataract.[2]
- Persistent leak from the thin area of conjunctiva overlying the bleb.
- Bleb infection. This can be blebitis (Fig. 12.3), a localised bleb infection, or endophthalmitis, if the infection spreads inside the globe. Endophthalmitis manifests as a painful red eye, with reduced visual acuity, and may be associated with hypopyon. Both blebitis and endophthalmitis require immediate referral to an ophthalmologist.
- Altered refractive error.
- Ptosis may occur, because positioning the eye in downgaze, plus holding the lids apart with a speculum during the operation, stretches the levator complex.

12.2.4 LONG-TERM IOP CONTROL FOLLOWING TRABECULECTOMY

This depends partly on what has happened to the eye before trabeculectomy and partly on other risk factors. Most patients who need trabeculectomy in the UK have received anti-glaucoma eye drops for 1–2 years prior to surgery. In a study comparing medical, laser and surgical management of POAG[3] 98% of patients who had a trabeculectomy when their glaucoma was diagnosed had an IOP of less than 21 mmHg 5 years later. However, in the Fluorouracil Filtration Surgery Study[4] (see section 12.2.5), only 26% of patients who had undergone previous intraocular surgery had a functioning trabeculectomy 5 years after their operation.

The following risk factors for failure of trabeculectomy have been identified:

- Previous cataract or glaucoma surgery – especially if the conjunctiva has been manipulated as part of the procedure.
- Prolonged treatment with anti-glaucoma eye-drops, especially sympathomimetics, e.g. dipivefrine (Propine). The impact of prior medical treatment on the outcome of trabeculectomy was investigated by Broadway et al in 1994.[5] For patients who received β-blockers preoperatively, the 6-month success rate of trabeculectomy was 93%; if β-blockers and pilocarpine were used preoperatively the 6-month success rate was 72%; if sympathomimetics were used in addition to β-blockers and pilocarpine, the 6-month success rate was 45%. Conjunctival biopsies taken from patients at the time of surgery revealed increased numbers of inflammatory cells in patients who were on topical triple-drop therapy of β-blocker, pilocarpine and sympathomimetic at the time of surgery or who had been on any type of eye drops for 3 or more years prior to surgery.
- Patients less than 40 years of age have a higher risk of failure than patients over the age of 40 years.
- There is a higher rate of failure in Afro-Caribbean patients compared with white patients.[6-8]
- Uveitis prior to trabeculectomy.[9]
- Neovascular glaucoma.[10]

12.2.5 WOUND HEALING IN FILTRATION SURGERY

Trabeculectomy failures occur mainly because of subconjunctival wound healing or fibrosis. Fibroblasts in the conjunctiva and Tenon's capsule are

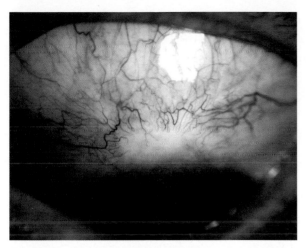

Fig. 12.4 A scarred trabeculectomy site. The wound healing response has caused scarring of the conjunctiva resulting in a flat, non-draining bleb.

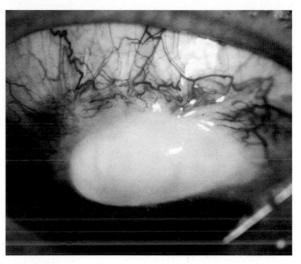

Fig. 12.5 A thin avascular bleb produced by using intraoperative 5-fluorouracil. Conjunctival inflammation surrounds the bleb.

responsible for the production of fibrin, i.e. scar tissue. The associated conjunctival scar blocks aqueous movement around the edges of the scleral flap (Fig. 12.4). The cell that is principally involved is the fibroblast, which produces the scar tissue. Antimetabolites, which were originally developed as anticancer drugs, are used to inhibit scarring that occurs in wound healing.

5-Fluorouracil

5-Fluorouracil (5-FU) can be applied intraoperatively. A sponge soaked in 5-FU is placed between the sclera and conjunctiva for 3–5 minutes before the scleral flap is made. The drug can also be applied postoperatively through subconjunctival injection. 5-FU inhibits fibroblasts without killing significant numbers of these cells. However, the use of 5-FU produces blebs with thin conjunctival roofs that can leak (Fig. 12.5), predisposing the patient to hypotony, blebitis and endophthalmitis. Multiple injections of 5-FU may lead to an epithelial keratopathy, characterised by pain and blurring of vision, which is usually reversible. In the Fluorouracil Filtration Surgery Study (FFSS),[4] patients with previous intraocular surgery who needed a trabeculectomy were randomised to receive either 21 postoperative injections of 5-FU over 2 weeks or placed in a control group who received no injec-

tions. At 5 years postoperatively, 49% of those who received 5-FU were successful, while the success rate of the control group was 26%. However, visual acuity was significantly worse in the early postoperative stages due to the reversible keratopathy in the 5-FU group. In addition, late-onset bleb leaks were more frequent in the 5-FU group (9%) than in the controls (2%).

Mitomycin C

This very powerful antimetabolite can only be applied intraoperatively on a sponge. Mitomycin C kills fibroblasts and produces very thin avascular blebs. There is a greater risk of hypotony, bleb leaks and endophthalmitis with mitomycin than with 5-FU.

For patients identified as being at significant risk of trabeculectomy failure, surgeons choose the metabolite that increases the chances of surgical success while not posing too great a risk of adverse reactions to the drug.

12.2.6 DRAINAGE TUBES, IMPLANTS AND SETONS

These are used in cases when one or two trabeculectomies with antimetabolites have failed.

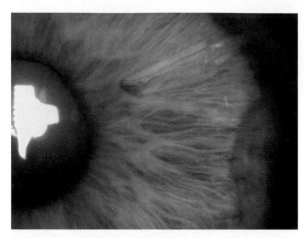

Fig. 12.6 A tube in the anterior chamber allows aqueous to leave the eye. The fluid collects posteriorly in the subconjunctival space.

Occasionally they are used in neovascular glaucoma as a primary procedure. The commonest device in use is the Molteno Tube (Fig 12.6). This surgery represents a more difficult operation compared with trabeculectomy. The principle is that the tube shunts aqueous from the anterior chamber through the sclera to a subconjunctival area overlying the posterior sclera. The scleral end of the tube is attached to an explant, which stimulates fibrosis around it, but the explant prevents conjunctiva adhering to sclera where aqueous leaves the tube.

One complication of drainage tubes is hypotony. Aqueous flows around the site where the tube penetrates the sclera to enter the anterior chamber. It is possible that too much aqueous will flow along the tube itself, leading to a lowering of IOP. Some devices are provided with valves that attempt to prevent this excessive flow occurring. Other complications resulting from drainage tubes include hyphaema, suprachoroidal haemorrhage, visual loss, and diplopia caused by the size of the explant and its placement close to the insertions of the recti muscles. In addition, there may be tube blockage with portions of the iris or vitreous in aphakic eyes, the tube may rub against the corneal endothelium, or the tube may migrate.

12.3 NON-PENETRATING GLAUCOMA SURGERY

This term refers to a surgical technique that includes some of the features of trabeculectomy but which does not involve removing the internal trabeculum. It covers two techniques: deep sclerectomy and viscocanalostomy. Both involve the creation of a scleral flap, however unlike a trabeculectomy no sclerostomy is created. Thus the anterior chamber is not entered. It is postulated that this results in fewer postoperative complications such as hypotony, inflammation, and shallow anterior chamber.

12.3.1 DEEP SCLERECTOMY

A one-third thickness limbal-based scleral flap is dissected and reflected forward. A block of deeper sclera is then dissected so that only a thin layer of sclera lies over the anterior choroid. The block is excised in such a way that the remaining sclera continues into the cornea exposing Schlemm's canal and Descemet's membrane. Aqueous can then be seen to ooze through the thin trabeculo-Descemet's membrane. Some surgeons then suture a collagen implant into the space created by excising the deep block. The scleral flap is sutured back into position over the implant and the conjunctiva repositioned. Aqueous is thought to leave the eye through subconjunctival and suprachoroidal routes.[11] The space created by excising the block of deep sclera, and maintained by the implant, is thought to act as a fluid reservoir.

12.3.2 VISCOCANALOSTOMY

Again a one-third thickness scleral flap is created; this is followed by the dissection of a deeper scleral flap to leave a thin layer of sclera and Descemet's. Before the deeper flap is excised Schlemm's canal is de-roofed and high-viscosity viscoelastic is injected into the exposed ends of the canal. The injection is thought to dilate Schlemm's canal and its connection with aqueous veins. Once the deeper scleral flap has been excised the superficial flap is sutured back into position and viscoelastic injected under the flap. Conjunctiva is then resutured over the sclera. The technique is postulated to work as in deep sclerectomy by allowing aqueous to move through the trabeculo-Descemet's membrane. It collects in the subscleral space before passing suprachoroidally, subconjunctivally, and into the now dilated Schlemm's canal.

12.3.3 RESULTS OF NON-PENETRATING SURGERY

Initial reports of both techniques have suggested that they are capable of lowering IOP.[11–13] However several trials have now randomised patients to either non-penetrating surgery or trabeculectomy. In two studies trabeculectomy produced a lower IOP[14,15] whereas in the third there was no difference.[16] However in all three the rate of postoperative complications was lower in the non-penetrating surgery group.

Treatment options for closed angle glaucoma

Closed angle glaucoma occurs as a result of anatomical obstruction to normal flow of aqueous in the eye (see Chapter 2, Fig. 2.1). There are a variety of causes including:

- Pupillary block (more than 90% of cases)
- Lens-induced angle closure glaucoma (either intumescent or anterior subluxation)
- Malignant closed angle glaucoma
- Plateau iris closed angle glaucoma.

All finally force the peripheral iris against the TM. Treatment options include: medical treatment to lower pressure and clear the cornea; laser iridotomy, and trabeculectomy. Medical treatment is used initially and may or may not lower IOP (see Chapter 10).

In acute angle closure glaucoma there is an abrupt rise in IOP that frequently produces an oedematous cornea. The initial treatment uses systemic acetazolamide plus topical antihypertensive agents to bring the pressure down. Pilocarpine is only used once the pressure starts to fall; it is felt that the iris is usually ischaemic at presentation and

therefore unresponsive to immediate pilocarpine. It is common to admit patients at this stage for management of their nausea and pain. As the pressure falls the peripheral cornea usually clears, allowing a laser iridotomy to be performed. The iridotomy is usually performed as soon as practicable since there is a high risk of eyes 'escaping' from miotic control, even if the IOP is initially well controlled. In chronic angle closure glaucoma the cornea is usually clear at presentation because the rise in IOP has been longstanding. Medical treatment is again given while arrangements are made to perform a laser iridotomy.

12.4 LASER IRIDOTOMY

Laser iridotomy creates a new pathway for aqueous to flow to the trabecular meshwork. The flow of aqueous into the anterior chamber opens up the angle, provided the angle is not sealed by peripheral anterior synechiae. The fellow eye is usually treated at the same time since it is at significant risk of angle closure.

The laser iridotomy technique is as follows. Clear the peripheral cornea if required. Apraclonidine (see Chapter 10, section 10.5.6) may be given before and after laser treatment to prevent IOP pressure spikes. Instil anaesthetic eye drops. A special laser contact lens with an eccentric focusing lens is used. If possible, the laser is applied to the base of the iris crypts, because the iris is thinner in this area. Argon or neodymium:yttrium aluminium garnet (Nd:YAG) lasers are equally effective, but Nd:YAG is more commonly used in the UK. Laser is applied to the iris between 11 o'clock and 1 o'clock, so that the upper lid covers the iridotomy. The operator can see when the laser penetrates the iris because a jet of aqueous accompanied by pigment flows forward through the iridotomy.

12.4.1 COMPLICATIONS OF LASER IRIDOTOMY

- Blurred vision
- Diplopia and glare, if the iridotomy is not covered by the upper lid

- Corneal damage
- Uveitis
- Raised IOP
- Haemorrhage/hyphaema
- Non-patent iridotomy
- Lens damage – rarely causes visual loss
- Retinal damage, though rare, may occur.

12.4.2 OUTCOME OF LASER IRIDOTOMY

In acute angle closure glaucoma there is often a rapid reduction in IOP, if a successful iridotomy is formed. In chronic angle closure glaucoma peripheral anterior synechiae, which have formed over a period of time due to the chronic close apposition of the iris to the angle, may prevent the angle from opening. Progressive peripheral anterior synechiae formation can reverse the initial successful outcome. Also iridotomies can close up, requiring repeat treatment.

12.5 SURGICAL IRIDECTOMY

This procedure is rarely performed today, and is reserved for those cases where laser treatment is ineffective, unavailable or not technically possible, or if laser iridotomy repeatedly blocks up. The technique is performed in an operating theatre under local or general anaesthesia. An incision is made in the cornea at 12 o'clock. The iris is prolapsed through the incision, and the iridectomy is cut with scissors. The iris is reposited, i.e. repositioned in the anterior chamber. The cornea is sutured.

12.6 CYCLOABLATIVE PROCEDURES

Cycloablative procedures are used on patients who have unmanageable glaucoma, poor visual prognosis, have had multiple operations, or who are unsuitable for surgery. Either infrared laser or cryotherapy is used to destroy the ciliary processes, thereby reducing aqueous production.

12.6.1 TRANS-SCLERAL CYCLOPHOTOABLATION

Laser burns are applied transconjunctivally through the sclera to the ciliary processes to reduce aqueous production. Both the Nd:YAG and semiconductor diode lasers are used. This technique is increasingly replacing cyclocryotherapy (see below). The technique for the Nd:YAG laser is either to use a contact fibreoptic probe placed on the limbus over the ciliary body or to use a non-contact method with the patient positioned on a slit-lamp. The laser is fired at the limbus and a contact lens may be used to position burns and prevent transpupillary treatment.

12.6.2 DIODE CYCLOPHOTOABLATION (CYCLODIODE)

This procedure uses a near-infrared laser with a wavelength of 810 nm. The laser passes through the sclera and is absorbed by melanin in the ciliary body and ciliary processes. The laser is applied using a fibreoptic probe. The technique is carried out under local or general anaesthesia with 50 burns applied over 360° of limbal area. The areas at 3 o'clock and 9 o'clock are spared to avoid the long posterior vessels and to prevent anterior segment ischaemia. Following surgery, topical steroids are prescribed for 1 week. Complications of cyclophotoablation include uveitis, an initial IOP spike, visual loss, conjunctival burns, and rarely phthisis.

12.6.3 CYCLOCRYOTHERAPY

The introduction of the cyclophotoablation/cyclodiode with its lower prevalence of complications has reduced the use of cyclocryotherapy. In this procedure a metal cryoprobe is connected via flexible tubing to a nitrous oxide powered cryounit which operates at a temperature of −80°C. The technique is as follows. The patient is given local or general anaesthesia. The probe is placed 1–1.5 mm behind the limbus and cooled. An ice ball forms around the probe in the tissues of the eye. The probe is turned off and allowed to warm up before it is moved. A single cryo lesion is made every hour for 6 hours. Steroid and atropine drops are pre-scribed afterwards along with anti-glaucoma medication.

Complications of cyclocryotherapy include pain and uveitis, both of which can be quite severe. In addition there may be hyphaema, choroidal detachment and phthisis (phthisis has been reported to have a prevalence as high as 22%).

Acknowledgement
Supported by the Medical Research Council (UK) grant no. G9330070.

References

1. Eendebak GR, Boen Tan TN, Bezemer PD. Long-term follow-up of laser trabeculoplasty. Doc Ophthalmol 1990; 75:203–214.

2. Collaborative Normal-Tension Glaucoma Study Group. The effectiveness of intraocular pressure reduction in the treatment of normal-tension glaucoma. Am J Ophthalmol 1998; 126:498–505.

3. Migdal C, Gregory W, Hitchings R. Long-term functional outcome after early surgery compared with laser and medicine in open-angle glaucoma. Ophthalmology 1994; 101:1651–1656.

4. The Fluorouracil Filtering Surgery Study Group. Five-year follow-up of the Fluorouracil Filtering Surgery Study. Am J Ophthalmol 1996; 121:349–366.

5. Broadway DC, Grierson I, O'Brien, et al. Adverse effects of topical antiglaucoma medication. II. The outcome of filtration surgery. Arch Ophthalmol 1994; 112:1446–1454.

6. Miller RD, Barber JC. Trabeculectomy in black patients. Ophthalmic Surg 1981; 12:46–50.

7. Berson D, Zauberman H, Landau L, et al. Filtering operations in Africans. Am J Ophthalmol 1969; 67:395–398.

8. Merritt JC. Filtering procedures in American blacks. Ophthalmic Surg 1980; 11:91–94.

9. Heuer DK, Parrish RK 2nd, Gressel MG, et al. 5-Fluorouracil and glaucoma filtering surgery. II. A pilot study. Ophthalmology 1984; 91:384–394.

10. Heuer DK, Parrish RK 2nd, Gressel MG, et al. 5-Fluorouracil and glaucoma filtering surgery. III. Intermediate follow-up of a pilot study. Ophthalmology 1986; 93:1537–46.

11. Chiou AG, Mermoud A, Hediguer SE, et al. Ultrasound biomicroscopy of eyes undergoing deep sclerectomy with collagen implant. Br J Ophthalmol 1996; 80:541–544.

12. Sunaric-Megevand G, Leuenberger PM. Results of viscocanalostomy for primary open-angle glaucoma. Am J Ophthalmol 2001; 132:221–228.

13. Stegmann R, Pienaar A, Miller D. Viscocanalostomy for open-angle glaucoma in black African patients. J Cataract Refract Surg 1999; 25:316–322.

14. Lüke C, Dietlein TS, Jacobi PC, et al. A prospective randomized trial of viscocanalostomy versus trabeculectomy in open-angle glaucoma: a 1-year follow-up study. J Glaucoma 2002; 11:294–299.

15. O'Brart DP, Rowlands E, Islam N, et al. A randomised, prospective study comparing trabeculectomy augmented with antimetabolites with a viscocanalostomy technique for the management of open angle glaucoma uncontrolled by medical therapy. Br J Ophthalmol 2002; 86:748–754.

16. El Sayyad F, Helal M, El-Kholify H, et al. Nonpenetrating deep sclerectomy versus trabeculectomy in bilateral primary open-angle glaucoma. Ophthalmology 2000; 107:1671–1674.

Chapter 13

Glaucoma co-management

Paul GD Spry

13.1 INTRODUCTION

Optometry is evolving, and there is little doubt that the wealth of knowledge gained by undergraduates in optometry and visual science, in particular regarding ocular pathology, is under-used. However, this situation has begun to change with the extension of the role of optometry into monitoring eye disease. The participation of optometrists in monitoring disease has been termed 'co-management' (also sometimes referred to as 'shared care'). In broad terms, co-management refers to selected groups of patients being reviewed by optometrists as part of a multidisciplinary collaboration with ophthalmologists and other eye care professions. The locus of co-management will vary according to local requirements, and in the context of chronic glaucoma, there appear to be no barriers to community monitoring; the Royal College of Ophthalmologists recognises that where it is not possible to provide an efficient, high quality hospital-based service, a co-management scheme may be introduced.

Any discussion of co-management schemes must begin with a formal definition of the concept. It seems appropriate that this should be taken from the document that prompted the self-review of the care systems that have, until recently, been the standard for care of glaucoma patients and those suspected of having glaucoma. This document, entitled 'Integrating Primary and Secondary Healthcare' was published by the National Health Service (NHS) Management Executive in 1991.[1] It encouraged community optometric participation in appropriate aspects of secondary healthcare, such as screening and review of diabetic eye disease, monitoring glaucoma, and through provision of low vision services. Shared care was defined as 'the active pursuit of high-quality, seamless care at every level across the primary and secondary arms of the (health) service'. There are many potential benefits of co-management schemes:

- *Seamless patient care.* The abolition of formalised referrals allows multidisciplinary free flow of patient information.
- *Multidisciplinary collaboration.* Co-management breaks down barriers between participating professionals, facilitating education and informed decision making, and enhancing patient care.
- *More effective use of resources.* Patients are stratified according to risk and are directed towards appropriate clinicians, optometric or ophthalmologic. This division of labour may permit patients with stable disease to be cared for by optometric co-management/shared care clinicians, and those with progressive disease to be seen swiftly by trained medical staff.
- *Local provision.* Co-management services may be located closer to patients' homes or places of work, making attendance easier and less stressful.
- *Achieving an effective balance between primary, secondary and community care.* Stable chronic disease requiring routine follow-up can be moved from busy outpatient departments to well-equipped and appropriately trained optometrists.

13.1.2 ATTRIBUTES OF EYE CONDITIONS SUITABLE FOR CO-MANAGEMENT

Although this chapter is concerned primarily with co-management for glaucoma patients and those suspected of having glaucoma, consideration should be given to factors that identify candidate eye conditions suitable for co-management provision. At a recent debate on Shared Care Services during the Royal College of Ophthalmologists' annual congress, it was suggested that presence of most or all of the following attributes assists in identification of appropriate eye conditions.[2]

High volume

Co-management/shared care schemes may be most efficient for ocular conditions that require a large number of patient appointments. Efficiency in this context refers to both freeing up considerable ophthalmologist time and ensuring that resources required for initiation of the scheme are rapidly offset by patient throughput. High-volume conditions are those with either moderate to high incidence, therefore presenting frequently, e.g. 'red eye', or lower prevalence but chronic nature, therefore requiring many review appointments over time, e.g. chronic glaucoma.

Diagnostic clarity

Co-management/shared care schemes are most likely to be successful where those sharing the care have high levels of concordance on all aspects of care. Conditions where debate may regularly occur on the essential issue of diagnosis should be avoided, as this leads to potential for disagreement over time, threatening the success of the scheme.

Clinical algorithms available or definable

Ocular conditions with well-established clinical practice patterns are highly amenable to co-management/shared care as those involved are most likely to agree on fundamentals of how the scheme should operate. Schemes will benefit from established algorithms for patient examination, clinically significant outcome measures, treatment interventions (timing and type), and care pathways. Clinical practice patterns based on published reports from clinical trials may be especially useful. In the context of chronic glaucoma, examples of algorithms used by major multicentre clinical trials include those of the Ocular Hypertension Treatment Study,[3,4] the Advanced Glaucoma Intervention Study[5,6] and the Collaborative Initial Glaucoma Treatment Study.[7]

13.2 FACTORS LEADING TO THE DEVELOPMENT OF CO-MANAGEMENT

In the context of ophthalmology, there is an increasing burden of treatable chronic eye disease within the Hospital Eye Service (HES) for which NHS reform could optimise service provision. Alongside diabetic eye disease, alternative strategies for monitoring primary open angle glaucoma (POAG) have become a subject of much interest. The causes of this may be grouped broadly into three categories: clinical factors, professional factors and the care environment.

13.2.1 CLINICAL FACTORS

■ Glaucoma causes considerable outpatient clinic loading. Routine examinations of POAG patients and those suspected of having glaucoma occupy up to 25% of consultant outpatient clinic time in the UK.

■ Poor outpatient clinic access. A survey of general practitioners (GPs) in Avon, completed by 76% of GPs in the area, showed that although 87% of respondents thought the quality of service provided by their local ophthalmology referral centre to be good, 85% felt that the quantity of service was inadequate.[8] Similar surveys in 15 other health authority areas revealed that in 10 of these, current access to ophthalmology services was viewed as a high priority for improvement.

■ Demography predicts an increased glaucoma burden. Countries within the developed world have ageing populations which will result in older people making up a significantly larger proportion of the population. Since the prevalence and incidence of POAG increase with age, more people will require treatment as time passes. The chronic nature of this disease necessitates lifelong follow-up. These factors will serve to produce annual increases in the number of glaucoma-related outpatient visits.

■ Enhanced disease detection will identify more glaucoma. Although optometrists are the primary source of referrals for possible POAG to the HES, a high percentage of POAG in the community remains undetected. Since the mid-1980s research has brought considerable progress in our understanding of the natural history of the disease, and in developing tests for POAG which have increased discriminatory power (i.e. high sensitivity and specificity) giving improved detection. Dissemination of this information has been active and widespread amongst ophthalmic healthcare professionals. Also, ophthalmic healthcare is fortunate to be an area of rapid evolution of instrumentation. The objectivity of current test design, particularly fully-automated perimetry and non-contact tonometry, makes these tests ideal for delegation to trained non-optometric support staff, allowing these tests to be carried out on those groups at risk of POAG without increasing the time the optometrist spends with the patient. It is inevitable in time that routine fundal imaging will also be performed by support staff, thereby allowing the clinician to simply scrutinise results from tonometry, visual field testing, and optic disc assessment, and act as a decision maker. More widespread use of this classic triad of tests, carried out using modern equipment, and supported by improved knowledge of optometrists of the disease process and referral criteria will produce a higher yield of previously undiscovered disease.

13.2.2 PROFESSIONAL FACTORS

■ Ophthalmologists are aware of the increasing burden of POAG upon the HES, and the need to address the problem. Many ophthalmologists feel that time they currently spend on routine monitoring of chronic disease could be channelled more efficiently into specialist tasks which they alone are able to perform, such as surgical procedures and the management of outpatients with more complex problems.

- Many optometrists would like to become involved in secondary healthcare. As routine examiners of the visual field, intraocular pressure (IOP) and optic discs, optometrists are familiar with the procedures fundamental to glaucoma follow-up. Therefore, many optometrists wish to see their role expand beyond pure 'case-finding' into areas such as the monitoring of POAG.[9,10]

- Other professionals, such as orthoptists and nursing staff, the traditional outpatient support staff, would also like to increase their clinical roles.

- The College of Optometrists launched a series of postgraduate diplomas for College registered optometrists in 1999. These qualifications provide accreditation of those with specialist background knowledge and skills appropriate for co-management. The original syllabus included a single certificate in glaucoma contributing towards the diploma in ocular conditions. A second glaucoma certificate was added in 2004, with emphasis on glaucoma monitoring. Optometrists with both certificates receive a diploma in glaucoma.

13.2.3 CARE ENVIRONMENT

- Modern NHS design makes co-management/shared care logistics relatively easy. The purchaser–provider climate developed within the NHS in the 1990s popularised the concept of 'units' of care. For example, it is commonplace for a primary care trust to buy a number of glaucoma outpatient visits at a specified NHS trust hospital on behalf of the GPs they represent. Such a system is easily applied to the purchase of services by care providers other than NHS trusts, such as glaucoma follow-up visits carried out by optometrists. If optometrists are recognised as providers of this care by the relevant professional bodies and an appropriate fee for each 'unit' can be agreed, there appears to be no logistical reason to prevent optometric involvement. Some optometrists already have 'provider-codes' allowing them to contract their services for specified tasks.

- NHS restructuring may prioritise co-management. As strategic health authorities and primary care trusts evolve they are becoming more interested in the primary care professions and are developing primary care services, including optometric involvement in co-management schemes. As a result, the policy of always purchasing services, e.g. glaucoma follow-up appointments, from hospitals may be relaxed, encouraging the purchase of care from local providers such as accredited optometrists.

- NHS sight test availability may be extended to further high-risk groups. Depending upon current government policy, the availability of 'free' sight tests to those at high risk, for example black people, will inevitably affect the number of referrals for suspected POAG, because more people will have an eye examination if they do not have to pay for it. The number of referrals for suspected glaucoma dropped dramatically (by around 16%) when the universal NHS sight test was removed in 1989, and it is likely that numbers rose with subsequent partial reintroduction (for those over 60 years) in 1999.

- NHS financial constraints make increases in the number of ophthalmologists working in the HES unlikely. The increased burden on the HES caused by POAG could be reduced by increasing the number of ophthalmologists. However, this is likely to be prohibitively expensive, and ophthalmology training levels may not be able to meet demand for staff.

13.3 CO-MANAGEMENT: SOLUTION TO THE PROBLEM?

A successful co-management scheme should benefit each patient by maintaining or improving the accessibility and/or quality of care,[11] and several possible models for the scheme could be adopted.

One model is to use non-ophthalmologists within the HES. Optometrists' knowledge and skill in detection of glaucoma places them in a strong position to fulfil this role. This approach has the benefit of allowing direct multidisciplinary contact and so may be a viable option. Although this model may work well in some hospitals, others simply do not have the physical space to accommodate extra clinicians, nor are there sufficient optometrists working within the NHS. This suggests a second model, using optometrists in a community-based environment, either alongside GPs or in their own practices. The latter option seems to be preferable since it utilises existing instrumentation and provides services close to where patients live.

13.3.1 TYPES OF CO-MANAGEMENT/ SHARED CARE SCHEME

There are several models of glaucoma co-management, in which the role and responsibilities of the optometrist can differ significantly.[12,13] One constant factor in all the current models is that, as stated by the Royal College of Ophthalmologists, the *ultimate* responsibility for the patient rests with the ophthalmologist.[11] Three main types of scheme can be identified as shown below.

Parallel care

- All tests are performed by the optometrist.
- Results are passed to the ophthalmologist for treatment decisions.
- All responsibility lies with the ophthalmologist, but they do not need to be in attendance when the tests are performed.
- Works well in community-based or hospital-based practice.

Co-managed or managed care

- The optometrist must decide whether the patient's condition is stable or progressive.
- The optometrist's decision is based on a protocol.
- The optometrist's responsibility has been described as 'direct' but not 'ultimate'.
- Ideally suited to community optometric practice.

True shared care

- Typically the optometrist works in the HES outpatient clinics with the ophthalmologist.
- The optometrist takes the decision-making role for the management of the patient.
- The ophthalmologist should be freely available for consultation with the optometrist.
- The optometrist must be familiar with ophthalmologists' practice and typically works to a protocol.
- The optometrist's role closely resembles that of an ophthalmological clinical assistant.

If there is proof that optometrists can be successful in monitoring disease, this may prompt future expansion of the optometric role within co-management schemes. Since the boundaries of the issues of responsibility remain the subject of some debate, it would seem sensible for optometrists to ensure that they have appropriate indemnity before joining a co-management scheme. Information on, and clarification of the issues concerning indemnity are available from the Association of Optometrists' website (http://www.assoc-optometrists.org).

13.4 THE TRIPARTITE DOCUMENT: A FRAMEWORK FOR SHARED CARE

Guidelines for the initiation of co-management/shared care schemes resulted from constructive negotiations between the Royal College of Ophthalmologists, The Royal College of General Practitioners and the College of Optometrists. In January 1996, these three parties published a set of general guidelines for the clinician about to enter shared care.[11] They provide an outline of the requirements of schemes and how they should be designed. A summary of the important points within these Tripartite documents follows. The reader is also referred to the documents themselves.

13.4.1 GENERAL FRAMEWORK

Participation in co-management/ shared care schemes

Participation should be by named individuals, not practices.

Local organisation

Schemes arising from the enthusiasm of local professionals should, upon reaching formal discussions, develop a local framework, for example a committee representing participating professions, and a point of contact. All potential participants should be consulted and the final scheme should be acceptable to all. Consultation and representation on management committees should extend beyond the eye care professions and involve administrative funding bodies and patient interest groups. Local optometric committees (LOCs) are the usual forum for local discussion among optometrists, and LOCs can play a key role in the design and management of co-management schemes.

Protocols

A description of the local co-management/shared care service, including aims and objectives, should be produced. Procedures, rules and instructions should be agreed upon, clearly stated and adhered to at all times. A formal protocol of precise clinical requirements and specified clinical responsibility at each point within the scheme should be clearly stated.

Training

Further and continuing education will be required to ensure all participants are up-to-date with modern concepts regarding the disease process, its management, and relevant clinical techniques. Arrangements for the training of participants should be incorporated into the protocol.

Review and audit

Mechanisms should exist to review objectively the efficiency and effectiveness of the scheme, and these can be used to identify educational needs.

Funding

Funding for schemes comes from the commissioners of the service, who are usually the primary care trust or its equivalent. Local contracts could be established with individual optometrists to provide designated services.

13.4.2 FRAMEWORK FOR PATIENTS WITH STABLE GLAUCOMA AND OCULAR HYPERTENSION

1. *Suitable patients.* A patient's condition should be stable with unchanged treatment for 2 years.
2. *Equipment standardisation.* High quality, standardised equipment is imperative. All participants should agree upon standards so results are reproducible between the HES and the optometric co-management practitioner (see Table 13.1).
3. *Training.* Participating optometrists should be trained to an agreed standard. Some of this may be provided within local HES clinics under supervision by the consultant ophthalmologist who may then assess the standards reached by all participants.

Table 13.1 **Details of equipment standardisation***

Tonometry	Applanation tonometry recommended
Funduscopy	Direct ophthalmoscopy acceptable although binocular indirect ophthalmoscopy is recommended (90D or 78D lenses)
Optic disc assessment	Appearance reported in a standard fashion supported by a written description and/or a drawing
Visual field analysis	Ideally, optometric instrumentation should be identical to that of the Hospital Eye Service. Appropriate test strategies for the individual patient must be agreed

* After Tripartite Document.[11]

4. *Communication.* Full reports should be sent from the ophthalmologist to the GP and co-management optometrist upon the entry of a patient into a co-management scheme. Both the GP and ophthalmologist should be informed of the results at each patient visit. This information should include details of new symptoms, compliance with treatment and clinical results.

5. *Follow-up.* Co-management assessments may take place at 6, 9 or 12 months, tailored to each patient, and the facility for ophthalmological review every 2 years should be considered.

6. *Re-referral.* Any signs of glaucomatous progression should produce re-referral to the ophthalmologist. Such signs include symptoms attributable to significant visual loss, IOP greater than the patient's agreed target pressure, deterioration of the visual field or change in the appearance of the optic disc.

13.5 VALIDATION

13.5.1 BRISTOL SHARED CARE GLAUCOMA STUDY

Because shared care represents a departure from routine clinical practice, it is important to ensure that it is validated, and explicitly provides a quality of care that is at least of equal standard to current practice patterns. In the context of glaucoma co-management, robust evidence for this and other aspects of co-management is available from a randomised controlled trial, the Bristol Shared Care Glaucoma Study.[13–19] This prospective investigation assessed community-based optometric managed care. The study revealed that around 23% of individuals passing through HES glaucoma clinics (around 6% of the total outpatient load) were eligible for optometric co-management according to defined recruitment criteria (Table 13.2). At each 6-monthly co-management follow-up appointment, around 20% of patients within the scheme were re-referred, following comparison of test results with baseline data (see Table 13.3 for criteria), for suspected glaucomatous instability. Four key aspects critical to the success of co-management were investigated.

Table 13.2 **Bristol Shared Care Glaucoma Study recruitment criteria***

Inclusion criteria	Exclusion criteria
Glaucoma suspects	Unstable glaucoma
Stable: primary open angle glaucoma; pigmentary glaucoma; pseudoexfoliative glaucoma	Other glaucomas: normal tension glaucoma; secondary glaucomas; narrow angle glaucomas
Snellen acuity of 6/18 or better in both eyes	Coexisting ocular pathology
Aged 50 years or over	Extensive field loss (>66/132 points missed at any suprathreshold increment on Henson suprathreshold examination)
Ability to cooperate with examinations	

*After Spencer et al.[14]

Measurement reliability

For applanation tonometry, binocular indirect ophthalmoscopic optic disc assessment, and Henson 132-point threshold-related suprathreshold visual field analysis, measurements made by glaucoma-trained optometrists were found to be as reliable and valid as those made within the traditional HES outpatient environment.[16,17]

Equality of outcomes

Over a 2-year longitudinal follow-up period, there were no marked or statistically significant differences in clinical outcomes (measures of the visual field, cup-to-disc ratio or IOP) between patients followed up in the hospital eye service or by community optometrists.[18]

Patient satisfaction

Information was collected on the time patients spent at appointments, their travelling costs and their perception of service quality. This revealed that patients were significantly more satisfied with

Table 13.3	Re-referral criteria used by the Bristol Shared Care Glaucoma Study*	
Test	**Glaucoma suspect**	**Glaucoma patient**
IOP	≥ 30 mmHg	≥ 24 mmHg
Optic disc	Vertical cup/disc ratio increase of ≥ 0.20 *or* disc haemorrhage	Vertical cup/disc ratio increase of ≥ 0.20 *or* disc haemorrhage
Visual field	'Defect' on Henson index of suspicion	Increase in number of points missed at any suprathreshold increment by ≥ 4 (mean increase of two tests)[†]

* After Spencer et al.[14]

[†] An increase of ≥ 7 missed points with a 132-point test initiated a second test. The mean result was compared with baseline measurements.

a number of aspects of care provided by community optometrists compared with the HES. This was particularly evident for waiting times, where periods of at least 30 minutes were exceeded in 50% of HES attendances compared with only 1% for optometric practice.[16]

Cost analysis

Objective determination of the costs of hospital and optometric practice is complex: a simple comparison is inappropriate. A full discussion of this issue is beyond the scope of this chapter and for a detailed discussion the reader is referred to Coast et al.[15] This paper is the only available detailed cost analysis of a co-managed scheme for glaucoma. Briefly, a variety of different approaches to cost analysis reveal that with an optometrist performing all investigations, community optometric co-management is unlikely to be the least expensive option. For equal (6-month) follow-up intervals, annual cost per patient (1994 prices) for optometric monitoring varied from £68.98 to £108.98 compared with £24.16 to £99.92 for the HES.[13,15] It should be stressed that these are actual costs and do not represent a recommendation for a service fee. Delegation to non-optometrically qualified staff of certain tasks may considerably reduce these figures for optometric monitoring, enhancing optometric competitiveness.

Although the Bristol Study therefore provides evidence that supports the feasibility of glaucoma co-management, the success of local schemes depends upon their validation, which should also demonstrate that a satisfactory care standard has been achieved. Validation for individual schemes may be gained using the audit process. Audit of scheme structures (e.g. equipment, training) and processes (e.g. all patients seen, follow-up intervals) may be beneficial early in the course of the scheme, with regular clinical audit to monitor decision-making thereafter.

13.6 SOME EXAMPLES OF CO-MANAGEMENT/SHARED CARE SCHEMES

The following examples of schemes describe different approaches to co-management/shared care, each of which is tailored to the requirements of the area in which it operates.

13.6.1 GLASGOW REVIEW CLINIC

This model of parallel care is based within the HES, uses existing optometric staff and facilities, and stratifies patients by risk. In the Glasgow Review Clinic, patients referred for ophthalmological assessment and found to be at low risk of developing glaucoma were discharged, whereas those requiring close supervision but not warranting ophthalmologist attention were placed within the shared care review clinic, being seen at 6–12 month intervals. This group of patients included both patients with POAG and those suspected of having glaucoma. A standard test protocol was used, including questions about compliance with treatment. Re-referral to the ophthalmology clinic was available if indicated, otherwise patient notes were reviewed annually by their consultant.

The results of an audit at 3 years showed that 50% of patients in the review clinic had POAG, 30% were suspected of having glaucoma with the remainder having angle closure or other types of glaucoma. Over 50% of attendees were on treatment. Over a 2-year period, the re-referral rate was 41%, although around half of these were classified as being over-cautious and were not confirmed as cases of instability.

The benefits of this scheme include the minimisation of the logistical problems of personnel, training, equipment and assessment standardisation. Interdisciplinary communication and patient follow-up are readily organised, even in the event of non-attendance. A major disadvantage is the administrative burden borne by the ophthalmologist in the annual assessment of case notes.

13.6.2 BRISTOL EYE HOSPITAL SHARED CARE DEPARTMENT

This model represents an example of true shared care. This clinical service development demonstrated a commitment to shared care as an accepted method of glaucoma care provision by establishment of an independent hospital department in 2000. Optometrists in the Shared Care Department are trained by formalised apprenticeship, using an 'in-house' training period spent gaining hands-on experience with glaucoma subspecialist consultants. Completion of training is assessed by comparison of a number of clinical measures and decisions. Trained 'shared care practitioners' work alongside consultant ophthalmologists in both new and follow-up outpatient glaucoma patient clinics. Practitioners have a high degree of autonomy, making all test-appropriate clinical measurements and taking clinical decisions regarding glaucoma status for follow-up patients, and discussing any uncertainties and treatment intervention requirements with the consultants. For new patients, practitioners make all baseline test measurements and make a provisional diagnosis and treatment suggestion, overseen on a case-by-case basis by the consultant.

At the present time, in excess of two-thirds of glaucoma follow-up in Bristol is performed by optometrists. Because of the need to seek approval for all treatment changes, limited prescribing status has been obtained for specified anti-glaucoma medications using a Patient Group Direction NHS procedure.

13.6.3 COMMUNITY BASED CO-MANAGEMENT SCHEMES

Schemes have been established in many areas, including Bradford, Burton, Humberside, Hull, South Staffordshire and West Kent. All follow the frameworks given in section 13.4, though each scheme has its local variations. Details of all these schemes are available on the Association of Optometrists (AOP) website. On its website the AOP has provided an excellent resource on co-managed care for the optometric profession, with sections on 'Getting involved in co-management', 'Contracts, indemnity and fees', schemes for the management of glaucoma, cataract, diabetes, etc. A copy of the joint AOP, College of Optometrists and Federation of Ophthalmic and Dispensing Opticians (FODO) document 'Guidance on Transparency in Co-Management' is available on this site, and tackles important clinical governance issues, notably ensuring that there is fairness and transparency in how schemes are established and how participating optometrists are selected.[20]

13.7 SUMMARY

Co-management is an exciting response to a variety of factors generating optometric involvement in aspects of secondary care of chronic eye disease. It is likely that participation in a scheme will play an increasing part in the workload of optometrists who elect to become involved. The new and interesting nature of the responsibilities co-management entails will increase and diversify optometrists' clinical abilities and role. Considerable information about initiating and designing a scheme is available in the form of the tripartite guidelines and from existing examples of co-management/shared care schemes. These should provide the potential participant with a framework for a scheme which may be tailored to meet the demands unique to their area. Development of optometric anti-glaucoma medication prescribing either within NHS Trusts or more widely may further extend the scope of co-management/ shared care schemes.

Acknowledgements

The author extends thanks to Mr JF Giltrow-Tyler, MCOptom, and Mr JM Sparrow, FRCOphth, for their valuable input to this manuscript.

References

1. NHS Executive. Integrating Primary and Secondary Healthcare. London: National Health Service; 1991.
2. Sparrow JM (chairman), Spry PGD, Murdoch I. Shared Care Debate. Royal College of Ophthalmologists Annual Congress, Birmingham, England, 2003.
3. Gordon MO, Beiser JA, Brandt JD, et al. The Ocular Hypertension Treatment Study: baseline factors that predict the onset of primary open-angle glaucoma. Arch Ophthalmol 2002; 120:714–20; discussion 829–830.
4. Gordon MO, Kass MA. The Ocular Hypertension Treatment Study: design and baseline description of the participants. Arch Ophthalmol 1999; 117:573–583.
5. AGIS Investigators. The Advanced Glaucoma Intervention Study (AGIS): 1. Study design and methods and baseline characteristics of study patients. Control Clin Trials 1994; 15:299–325.
6. AGIS Investigators. The advanced glaucoma intervention study (AGIS): 7. The relationship between control of intraocular pressure and visual field deterioration. Am J Ophthalmol 2000; 130:429–440.
7. Musch DC, Lichter PR, Guire KE, et al. The Collaborative Initial Glaucoma Treatment Study: study design, methods, and baseline characteristics of enrolled patients. Ophthalmology 1999; 106:653–662.
8. Hicks NR, Baker IA. General practitioner views of options of health services available to their patients. Br Med J 1985; 302:991–993.
9. Various authors. Shared care in glaucoma and ocular hypertension. Highlights of a national conference held at Coombe Abbey, Binley, June 1996. Kingston-upon-Thames: Medicom (UK) Publ Ltd; 1996.
10. Giltrow-Tyler F. Sharing the responsibility. Optician 1993; 206:15–17.
11. Royal College of Ophthalmologists, Royal College of General Practitioners, College of Optometrists. Shared care for patients with stable glaucoma and ocular hypertension. General framework for shared care schemes. London: Royal College of Ophthalmologists; 1996.
12. Giltrow-Tyler F. Shared care. Optometry Today 1996: 26–30.
13. Spencer IC, Coast J, Spry PG, et al. The cost of monitoring glaucoma patients by community optometrists. Ophthalmic Physiol Opt 1995; 15:383–386.
14. Spencer IC, Spry PG, Gray SF, et al. The Bristol Shared Care Glaucoma Study: study design. Ophthalmic Physiol Opt 1995; 15:391–394.
15. Coast J, Spencer IC, Smith L, et al. Comparing the costs of monitoring glaucoma patients: hospital ophthalmologists versus community optometrists. J Health Serv Res Policy 1997; 2:9–25.
16. Gray SF, Spencer IC, Spry PG, et al. The Bristol Shared Care Glaucoma Study – validity of measurements and patient satisfaction. J Public Health Med 1997; 19:431–436.
17. Spry PGD, Spencer IC, Sparrow JM, et al. The Bristol Shared Care Glaucoma Study: reliability of community optometric and hospital eye service test measures. Br J Ophthalmol 1999; 83:707–712.
18. Gray SF, Spry PG, Brookes ST, et al. The Bristol shared care glaucoma study: outcome at follow up at 2 years. Br J Ophthalmol 2000; 84:456–463.
19. Spry PGD, Sparrow JM. Can optometrists monitor glaucoma? A review of the Bristol shared care glaucoma study. Optometry Pract 2001; 2:47–56.
20. Association of Optometrists, College of Optometrists, and Federation of Ophthalmic and Dispensing Opticians. *Guidance on Transparency in Co-Management*. 2004. Available at: www. assoc-optometrists.org

Index